Published by
Wrathall Publishing
Lancaster

First Published
May 2014

Website:
www.ibsrecovery.co.uk

Designed by
Dean Chillmaid @ Spacehopper Design
www.spacehopperdesign.co.uk

Printed in Malta on behalf of
Latitude Press Limited

DEDICATION

This book is dedicated to the memory of my father

James Stephen Wrathall (Jim)

Who was a diabetic, and died after a series of strokes prior to the writing of this book.

I am now convinced from his history, over the first 42 years of his life, and in particular, his diet, which in the main consisted of large quantities of sugar, wheat, and dairy, was a, or, the causal factor in creating the conditions, which led to the onset of his affliction, namely type one insulin dependant diabetes?

QUALIFICATIONS

This book has been written by myself, John Stephen Wrathall, ND, Naturopathic doctor, herb (dip).

All the advice in this book is as a result of years of experimenting at a personal level, and with others who were freely willing to adopt this recovery programme, after themselves having years of undiagnosed stomach and bowel problems.

I have studied naturopathic principles for four years, at Manchester university, and have gained a ND (naturopathic medicine diploma) which involved the study of many different systems, modalities, and methods of treatment, these included the following.

Medical subjects:
Cardiovascular system
Musculoskeletal system
Lymphatic system
Endocrine system
Skin
Respiratory system
Urinary system and electrolytes
Digestive system
Reproductive system
Nervous system
Oncology
Infectious diseases
Immune system
Examination methods
Allergology
Medical terminology
Case taking
Anatomy and physiology
Pharmaceutical practice

Other modalities studied:
Tissue salts
Traditional Chinese medicine
Ayuervedic medicine
Herbal medicine
Auricular acupuncture
Bach flowers
Iridology
Nutrition and its affects on health

Clinical hours
450 clinical hours treating patients under supervision have also been completed before the qualification was obtained.

CONTENTS

1. Dedication   2

2. Qualifications   3

3. Introduction   10
Cut Out List Of Foods That Cannot Be Eaten   14
Cut Out List Of Foods That Can Beaten   15

4. Acknowledgment   17

5. Symptoms Relating To Intolerance   18
List Of Symptoms   18
Clues In Younger Years   23
Teens And Early Twenties   24
More Recently   25
The Mid Life Reprieve   26
Parents, Brothers And Sisters, Sons And Daughters   27
Diary Of Foods And Reaction Chart   28
Reaction Chart   30
Diary   32
Intense Reaction   37
Other Observed Symptoms   38
Yeast Overgrowth   40
Helicobacter Pylori   40

6. Foods That Cannot Be Eaten   42
Wheat Products   42
Dairy Products   44
Soya Products / Tofu   45
Other Intolerance Foods   45

7. Foods That Can Be Eaten   46
Wallchart List   48
Greens   50
Bio Yoghurt   50
Meats And Protein   50
Diet Relating To The Recovery Programme   50
Self Help   51
Sugary Products = Feeling Very Hungry.   51
Other Reactions   52
Possible Foods For Each Meal   53
Foods For Breakfast: 53
Foods For Lunch: 54
Some Of My Recipes   57
Breakfast Recipes   57
Lunch Recipes   60
Dinner Recipes   62
What Can You Eat After Full Recovery?   70

8. What Can I Drink?   **70**
Alcohol   70
Wine   70
Tea And Coffee   70
Orange Juice And Oranges   70
Fizzy Drinks   70
Soya Milk   70
Daily Drinks   70
Water (At Least 1 Litres A Day)   71
Alcoholic Drinks   73
Motto; "Think Before You Drink"   73
Soups Or Broths As A Drink   74

9. The Recovery Programme   **76**
Getting Started   76
The First Month   76
The Second Month   77
3 To 12 Months   78
12 To 16 Months   79
16 To 24 Months   79
24 Months On   81

10. Acknowledgement   **83**

11. What Happens In Recovery?   **84**
Initial Advice   84
First Two Months   85
2 To 12 Months   86
12 To 24 Months   87
Headache   88
Acid Reflux   88
Hunger   88
Water   89
Bloated Appearance   89
Weight   89
Tiredness   89
Exhaustion   89
Aching Muscles, Back, Joints   89
Eyes   89
Gallstone Indicators   90
Helicobacter Pilori   90
Anxiety And Memory   91
Celiac   91
Tingling Numbness And Dead Limbs   91
Urine Colour   92
Kidney Flush   92
Gallbladder And Liver Flush   92
Yeast Overgrowth   92
Athletes Foot, Toenails   92

Temper 92
Feeling Cold 93
Lines On Fingernails 93
Dry Patches Of Skin, Lips, Skin Palpitations, Itching 93
Impotency 94
Stool Colours 94
Finally 95

12. Can You Eat Wheat Dairy And Other Products Again? **96**
Wheat Products 96
Dairy Products 97
Oats 98
Other Products And Receding Food Intolerance 98

13. What Happens To The Digestive Tract? **100**
The Mouth 102
The Stomach 102
The Small Intestine 103
Duodenum 103
Jejunum 103
Ileum 103
The Large Intestine 104
Ascending, Transverse, Descending And Sigmoid. 104
Rectum 104
Pertalsisis 104
Acid Reflux 106
Bowel Reactions 107
The Emerging Emergency State 108
Celiac Disease 109
Irritable Bowel Syndrome 110
The Emergency State 111
Observations 112
M.E, Yuppie Flue 114
The Crucial Key To Recovery 114
Digestive Tract Timing And I.B.S 115
The Liver And Gallstones 119
The Symptoms Of Gallstones 119
The Pancreas 125
The Dairy Connection 129
The Wheat Connection 130
The Sugar Connection 130
Summary 131
Associated Problems 131
Beriberi 134
Rickets 134
Scurvy 134

14. What's Wrong With Wheat Products? **136**
Observations 136
Flour And Bread, Oats And Corn 137

Modern Yeasts   139
Anaemia, Iron And Calcium   139
Other Possible Problems   141
Alternatives To Modern Wheat   142
Experiment   143

15. Acknowledgment   **147**

16. What's Wrong With Dairy Products?   **148**
Problems With Dairy Products   148
Dairy And Gluten Connection   151
Reactions   152
Conclusion   152

17. Acknowledgement   **155**

18. What's Wrong With Carbohydrate?   **156**
Digestive Problems And Sugar   156
The Liver And Sugar   158
Carbohydrate And Diabetes   158
History And Carbohydrate   160
Conclusion   160

19. Helicobacter Pylori   **162**
Warning   162

20. Yeast Overgrowth Or Candida Albicans   **164**
What Is Yeast Overgrowth / Candida Albicans?   164
Intestinal Microbes And Health   165
What Causes Yeast Overgrowth   165
Treatment In Relation To Diet   167
Killing Off Yeast Overgrowth   169
Aids To Killing Yeast Overgrowth   170
Foods To Be Avoided With Yeast Overgrowth   171
Athletes Foot, Thick Toenails, Bacteria   172

21. Acknowledgement   **174**

22. Toxins And Oxidants   **178**
Which Products Are Toxic And Oxidising?   179
Fried Foods   179
Coffee   179
Smoking   181
Alcohol   181
Sunlight   181
Fumes   181
Toxic Overload   182
Sensitivity To Toxins And Oxidants   183

23. Time, Memory, Stress And The Mind   **184**
Time   184
Memory And The Mind   184
Stress And The Common Bile Duct   186

The Digestive Tract And The Mind 187
Food And The Mind 189

24. The Cold Phenomena 192
After Full Recovery 193

25. Exercise And Rest 196
Exercise 196
Rest 198
Observations 200

26. Vitamins And Minerals 202
Anaemia 203
Digestive Tract Reaction 204
Problems At The Molecular Level 206

27. Acknowledgement 208

28. History 212
The Wheat Connection 213
The Dairy Connection 214
Man's Environment 214
Water Consumption 217

29. The Kidney Cleanses 218
The Kidneys And Kidney Stones 218
When Do You Cleanse The Kidneys? 219
Symptoms 220
Causes 221
My Experience 222
Possible Reactions 222
The Beetroot Cleanse 223
The Herbal Cleanse 224
The Lemon Juice Cleanse 225
Warning 225
Conclusion And The Future 226

30. The Gall Bladder And Liver Flush 228
When Not To Flush 228
When Should You Flush? 229
Possible Symptoms Of Gallstones 230
Symptoms Of Becoming Blocked Between Flushes 233
My Experience 234
Minor Problems When Flushing 235
The Flush 236
What Is The Apple Juice Doing? 237
What Are The Epsom Salts Doing? 237
Why You Need To Lie On Right And Left Side's And Pull Your Knee Up? 237
The Gallbladder And Liver Flush 238
The First 5 Days 238
The Day After The Flush 239
Retrieving The Stones And Chaff 241

What Are You Looking For?   241
Shape Of Gallstones   242
What Can You Expect, And Find After A Flush?   242
Are They Gallstones   243
Conclusion   246

31. The In Depth Medical Explanations   248
Conventional Understanding   248
Mouth   248
Cephalic Phase Of Digestion   249
Stomach   249
Gastric Phase Of Digestion   250
Intestinal Phase Of Digestion   250
Breakdown And Absorption   251

32. Bowel Ph, Absolutely Vital   254
Bowel Ph   254

33. Digestive Compensation   256
Digestive Compensation Stage 1, Switching Between Normal Bowel And Constipation 256
Symptoms Of Digestive Compensation Stage 1   258
Digestive Compensation Stage 2, Switching Between Constipation And Loose Bowels 259
Symptoms Of Digestive Compensation Stage 2   261
Conditions Relating To Digestive Compensation Stage 2.   262
Digestive Compensation Stage 3, (The Emergency State), Permanent Loose Bowels 263
Symptoms Of Digestive Compensation Stage 3   265
Conditions Relating To Digestive Compensation Stage 3   266

34. Treatments   268
Conventional Treatment Protocols   268
Important Note   270

35. Observed Complications   272
Diabetes   272
Renin, Angiotensinogen, A.C.E, And Feeling Cold   274
Aldosterone Angiotensinogen And Feeling Weak, Me Symptoms   277
Sodium Potassium Pump   279
Conclusion   279
Rheumatic Symptoms   280
Blood Albumins   281
Plasma Cells And Immunity   282

36. Acknowlegement   285

37. Herbal Treatments   286
Herbs Used To Recover Systems?   286

38. Dare I Say It...   287
A Last Word   288
P.S   290

39.   Naturapathic Practitioners   292

40.   Thanks   293

41.   Index   294

INTRODUCTION

Hello

My name is John Wrathall

Welcome to the world of IBS and food intolerance.

I have three daughters, Charlotte Marie, and twins Kirsty Rose and Sophie Amelia. I have two brothers and one sister. I am the second in our family, the eldest being James, then myself, next Derek and lastly Janet. I now live with my wife Pam.

I have been prompted to write this book after years of visits to the doctors and hospital, to try and alleviate stomach and bowel problems.

In the latter days of my illness, and after investigations and biopsies to try and find the cause of my problems, I was told that I was borderline celiac, and would be treated as one, I also had Irritable Bowel Syndrome (I.B.S).

Later after my condition became worse, it was suggested that I could have developed M.E. (yuppie flu, or its official title, myalgic encephalomyelitis) I refused to believe that all the symptoms I had, which are listed in this book, could be untreatable conditions called celiac disease, IBS, or ME.

I thought to myself, something has to be causing this condition, it can't be something one just has to live with, this cannot be normal.

I began to think at the age of 42 and in the depths of my intolerance, that I would not get to retirement age at this rate, I felt so ill and worn out. I even began to think, maybe I've done too much manual work, I used to work seven days a week, and many of those were 16 hr days, have I worn my body out? I now know this not to be the case.

It seems to me that the medical profession use the term ME, Yuppie Flue, IBS as a pigeonhole to put people in, when there isn't a test to define a definite, definable, condition or illness. This leaves people like us in medical no mans land.

So I set about the task of trying to find out what was wrong with me, little knowing where it would lead me, and how long it would take to finally arrive at a reasoned answer.

In this book I will take you through a life history of the symptoms and eventual understanding of food intolerance, which I now know, affects a significant proportion of the population.

It appears that many of us do not have the digestive system to cope with prolonged ingestion of fortified flours, processed sugar and pasteurised dairy products, without developing digestive problems. I can now say with conviction that in almost all cases, if you are intolerant to dairy products you are also intolerant to wheat products and visa versa. The causal factor has been your over indulgence in mainly wheat gluten based products, and secondly dairy products and processed sugar throughout your lifetime.

The main problems as far as I can work out, are with the high gluten protein wheat-based, processed products. This will be your first and trigger intolerance.

The long-term consequences of ingesting too many of the aforementioned wheat dairy and sugar based foods, causes the digestive system, liver and pancreas to degrade, and may lead to other possible problems developing, such as gallstones, which in turn leads on to IBS (irritable bowel syndrome) and other conditions such as Celiac disease, ME, and even diabetes.

The aforementioned initially leads to liver efficiency problems, where the production and free flow of bile is impaired, impinging on the pancreas, and affecting the production of digestive enzymes and hormones.

Almost invariably if you are intolerant to wheat you are intolerant to dairy products, for the reasons explained in this book, and you will probably have yeast overgrowth, (Candida Albicans), also covered in this book.

This will not be a complicated in depth study of diet or the human anatomy, but a basic common sense approach to the modern diet, and how it affects modern man in what is now becoming an alien environment of processed foods and unnatural substances.

Most of the understanding, treatments, and dietary recommendations in this book, have been arrived at in the first instance, through personal experimentation on myself, and subsequently other people who fulfilled the same symptoms criteria as myself.

It was only after the very careful recording and analysis, and the reactions to the foods others and I ate or drank, that I began to unravel the common factors, and underlying causes of many people's food intolerances and related conditions. This is not to say that I have all the answers in what is a very complex, and as yet in the most part a little understood phenomenon.

It will not be an unaffordable diet but a practical everyday approach to the problem, which people can understand and follow.

But this I do know, there are elements in mainly wheat, and to a lesser degree dairy products and processed sugar, which if taken in too large a quantity over a lengthy period of time, are the trigger to intolerances and bowel disorders.

This I say with conviction and certainty after finding so many friends and acquaintances whom have patently gained intolerance to certain grains, or, more to the point, the way man has processed these grains, and to a degree dairy products.

In this book I have had to start with the assumption that you are very food intolerant where diet is concerned, and therefore in the early stages of recovery the diet is quite strict.

This is necessary to control severe food intolerance, and to relieve and address the inevitable bloating and inflammation in your bowel.

I would advise you to start from the assumption that you are very intolerant and work backwards, introducing small amounts of the intolerance foods as you progress in your recovery. However, wheat and dairy products should always be eaten in very small amounts, until any and all the necessary gallbladder and liver flushes have been completed.

I do not have a magic wand, and therefore you must understand that this is a two-year recovery programme, possibly even more if you are above 45 yrs old.
This is not a magic cure, but this I guarantee, if you fulfil the symptoms criteria and consequently adhere to the advice advocated in this book, I can be absolutely confident that you will regain full health and fitness. Therefore my assumptions and advice on this subject will be vindicated by your recovery.

So, if you decide after reading this book that you recognise yourself, in that you have all the classic symptoms of food intolerance, use this book as your bible of recovery. Read and digest it and become familiar with your condition and the associated problems. Use this recovery programme to the full, and give yourself your life back. Good luck and good health.

On the following pages are a list of foods that cannot be eaten, and a list of foods that can be eaten, you may want to cut these out and laminate them, and keep them on your kitchen wall, these lists are also in the chapters "foods that can be eaten", and "foods that cannot be eaten".

I have left the next page clean so you can use this to jot down any notes.

CUT OUT LIST OF FOODS THAT CAN'T BE EATEN

Wheat Products

- Barley
- Biscuits, [most kinds contain wheat]
- Bran and bran related cereals
- Breakfast cereals [some are malt flavoured, and some are wheat or bran, which will react with you, also contain small amounts of phytic acid]
- Bulgar [dried wheat]
- Cheese [some cheeses, especially yellow ones and mouldy ones may contain an element of wheat]
- Couscous [made from wheat]
- Curry mixes [may contain wheat flour]
- Dried meals [may contain wheat flour]
- Durum [a type of wheat]
- Flour [wholemeal, granary, brown, bread]
- Ginger beer [may contain wheat colouring]
- Gravy mixes [contain flour]
- Ice cream [some contain wheat starch]
- Lager, beer, stout [they potentially contain gluten]
- Lemonade [may contain wheat based colourings]
- Macaroni
- Millet
- Mustard powder [may contain wheat]
- Oats [similar gluten to wheat, may not affect all with this condition, contains phytic acid]
- Packet and tinned products [read labels all could have wheat starch or flour in them]
- Pasta [made from wheat]
- Peanuts [beware salted peanuts, they may contain wheat starch]
- Pills [they may be bound with a wheat-based product]
- Rice paper [some use wheat flour]
- Rye [contains gluten similar to wheat]
- Salad cream [contains vinegar and therefore possible wheat]
- Sausages [contain flour]
- Sauces [may contain wheat starch]
- Semolina [made from wheat]
- Soy sauce [fermented in wheat flower]
- Spaghetti [made from wheat]
- Spelt [similar protein, reacts in rare cases]
- Stock cubes and gravy cubes [may contain wheat]
- Starch [vegetable starch on processed or tinned food, this may be wheat starch]
- Toffees [some are dusted with wheat or have wheat starch]
- Tomato sauce [contains vinegar and possible wheat]
- Triticale
- Vinegar [contains wheat, rice vinegar is all right]
- Vitamin E pills [usually made from wheat]
- Wheat germ

Dairy Products

- Biscuits
- Butter
- Cakes [many contain dairy products, obviously they contain wheat too]
- Cheese
- Chocolate
- Creams and ice cream
- Margarine
- Milk
- Some confectionary
- Yoghurt [live yoghurt is all right and should be used, one or two servings every day, if very intolerant supplemant with pre and pro biotics and digestive enzimes.]

Soya Products:

Tofu - read all labels on products and avoid if Soya is present [meat could be Soya substitute]

OTHER INTOLERANCE FOODS:

Eggs - be wary of eggs in very early recovery.

Lemons, Limes - Very acidic, irritates stomach in early recovery.

Melons - This seems to be quite a common one.

Orange - Juices, Still orange, Fresh orange
People are usually intolerant until later into recovery.

Sesame Seeds - In extreme intolerance cases sesame seeds will react with you.

Stearic Acid - Beware of in tablets, if it's in a concentrated form it may react with you.

Tomatoes - In rare cases tomatoes may give you acid reflux in early recovery.

Cucumber - In very rare cases cucumber may react with you.

CUT OUT LIST OF FOODS THAT CAN BE EATEN

℞ # *Yeast overgrowth related foods. (eat in small amounts, and only after first two months)*
? *Oily foods. (eat in small amounts). All these foods may be eaten in normal amounts after full recovery.*

Almonds
Apples
Apricots #
Artichoke
Asparagus
Aubergine
Avocado pear
(small amounts at
first)
Bacon ?
Bamboo shoots
Bananas
Bean sprouts
Beans kidney
Beans runner
Beef, minced,
corned ?
Beetroot
Bilberries #
Blackberries #
Blackcurrants #
Bloater fish
Blueberries #
Brawn ?
Broccoli
Brussels sprouts
Buckwheat flour
Cabbage
Carrots
Cashew nuts
Cauliflower
Caviar
Celeriac
Celery
Cherries #
Chestnuts
Chicken (no skin)
Chickpeas
Chicory
Cockles
Coconut
Cod
Corn flour
Corn on the cob
Corn

Corned beef ?
Courgettes
Crab
Cranberries #
Crayfish
Cress
Crisps (plain rarely
as a treat)
Cucumber (be
wary of in early
recovery)
Currants #
Dates #
Dripping ?
Duck
Eels
Eggs
Endive
Fennel
Figs #
Flax seed
Fruit
(not oranges) #
Fruit salad (no
oranges) #
Gammon ham
(boiled)
Garlic (small
amounts at first)
Gherkins
Ginger
Goose
Gooseberries #
Grapefruit (in own
juice)
Grapes #
Greengage
Grouse
Haddock
Hake
Halibut
Ham ?
Hare ?
Hazelnuts
Heart ?

Herring ?
Honey #
Jams #
Kale
Ketchup ?
Kidney beans
Kidney ?
Kippers ?
Kiwi Fruit #
Lamb
Leek
Lemon (be
wary of in early
recovery)
Lemonade #
Lentils
Lettuce
Limes (be wary of
in early recovery)
Liver ?
Lobster
Loganberries #
Luncheon meat ?
Mackerel ?
Maize
Mango
Marrow
Mayonnaise ?
Meats red ?
Mint
Mung beans
Mushrooms #
Mussels
Mutton ?
Oil, Vegetable,
Olive etc ?
Okra
Olives ?
Onion (small
amounts at first)
Oranges (Be
wary of in early
recovery)
Oysters
Palm Hearts

Papaya
Parsley
Parsnips
Partridge
Peach #
Peanuts (beware
some brands
contain wheat)
Pear
Peas
Pepper
Peppermint (not
toffee mints)
Pheasant
Pilchards ?
Pine nuts
Pineapples (in
own juice)
Plaice
Plums #
Pomegranate
Pork ?
Potatoes
Prawns
Prunes #
Phsyllum seeds
Pumpernickel
Pumpkin & seeds
Rabbit ?
Radish
Raisins #
Raspberries #
Redcurrants #
Rhubarb
Rice (must be
brown)
Roe
Salad cream (very
small amounts)
Salmon
Sardines ?
Scallops
Seakale
Shellfish
Shrimps

Skate
Sole
Spinach
Spirulina
Sprats
Squash
Squid
Steak ?
Strawberries #
Suet ?
Sultanas #
Sunflower seeds
Swedes
Sweet corn
Sweet potato
Sweets #
Tomatoes (be
wary of early
recovery)
Tongue ?
Tripe ?
Trout
Tuna (drain brine
or sunflower oil)
Turbot
Turkey (no skin)
Turnip
Veal ?
Venison ?
Walnuts
Watercress
Whelks
Whitebait
Whiting
Yam
Yoghurt (Plain
Live only) one
serving every
day. If extremely
intolerant
supplement with
pro biotics and
digestive enzymes.
Instead of taking
live yoghurt

ACKNOWLEDGMENT

Since giving up wheat my years of
suffering with heartburn and indigestion.
disappeared within days.
Now eight months later and one stone and
three inches gone from my waist.
I feel much healthier and less lethargic

A Singleton

SYMPTOMS RELATING TO INTOLERANCE

Below is a list of symptoms, tick the boxes next to your symptoms, and then add up the numbers next to the boxes you have ticked to give you your score. Then refer to the notes at the end of the symptoms list; this will give you an indication of how far you have advanced in your intolerance.

The points system is just a rough guide, and more clues can be obtained if you read all the information in this chapter.

This chapter should aid you in deciding whether you have become a food intolerant.
This is as accurate a diagnosis as I can attain, without questioning you personally, in detail over a couple of hours.

Score		List Of Symptoms
1	☑	Aching back
4	☐	Aching joints, mainly aching knees and legs, shoulders and back, arthritic symptoms. [ache in right shoulder is a symptom of gallstones]
4	☐	Aching muscles
1	☑	Acne [as a teenager, and in later life in advanced cases. Not always a symptom]
2	☐	Anaemia, [lack of iron]
1	☑	Anxiety, worried by problems, easily stressed in advanced cases.
3	☑	Athlete's foot, mouldy dry skin between toes.
7	☑	Bloated appearance in face and puffy, possibly all over, [it's like every molecule in your body expands, possible water retention]
10	☐	Bloating stomach or lower abdomen
4	☐	Bruised feeling in stomach and lower abdomen, especially when tapped with fingers.
6	☑	Constipation
4	☐	Dead limb when sleeping [you should not get dead limbs or tingling at all when sleeping]
5	☐	Dermatitis Herpetiformis [red spots may be on dry patches of skin, itchy, don't come to a head, but bleed if scratched]
10	☑	Diarrhoea, loose bowels, or switching between loose bowels and constipation, light coloured pungent smelling and floaty stools
2	☐	Drained of energy on hot, clammy, summer days
4	☑	Dry bottom lip [symptom of gallstones]
4	☐	Dry patches of skin, possibly anywhere
4	☑	Emotional easily moved to tears, sharp tempered, snappy, but not necessarily bad tempered.

Score	List Of Symptoms
1 ☐	Eyes full of mucous in a morning,
2 ☐	Eyes gritty
6 ☐	Eyes sensitive to bright sunlight or car headlights, makes you squint,
1 ☐	Feeling unsteady and walking off to one side, usually right [in advanced cases, usually with hypoglycaemia, low blood sugar]
1 ☐	First breath after sleep you can feel lungs expand and gurgle slightly [advanced condition]
3 ☐	Flu like feeling [mild]
4 ☐	Gnawing, cramping feeling in stomach [symptom of helicobacter pylori]
1 ☐	Gums ache and bleed, especially when cleaning teeth
2 ☐	Haemorrhoids (piles)
1 ☐	Head feeling pressured, blown up [possibly high blood pressure]
4 ☐	Headaches [not all the time but regularly]
2 ☐	Heavy limbs
1 ☐	Hypoglycaemia [low blood sugar, in extreme cases, indication of gallstones]
3 ☐	Inability to put on weight, or weight loss (sufferers with celiac condition)
2 ☐	Irritability, slightly snappy but not necessarily bad tempered.
5 ☐	Itching all over [not all the time but occasionally]
2 ☐	Itchy rectum
2 ☐	Lack of breath, soon out of breath
2 ☐	Lack of self-motivation
2 ☐	Lack of sex drive [possible impotency in males]
4 ☐	Light headed, easily faint.(in advanced cases)
1 ☐	Lost sense of thirst [in rare cases, not all together but you never feel really thirsty, sign of gall stones]
5 ☐	Often tired in daytime.
2 ☐	Oily skin on face especially around bridge of nose [gallstone symptoms]
2 ☐	Pain in back after sleeping which is felt for 2-3 hours after rising. [symptom of Gallstones in advanced cases]
4 ☐	Pain under right hand ribcage and running around right hand side, and possibly under right hand shoulder blade [gallstone symptoms]
1 ☐	Roseacea [red cheeks and hot face, yeast overgrowth and sugar related]
1 ☐	Sensitive to car fumes, dust, detergents, smoke

Score	List Of Symptoms
3 ☐	Sinuses fluey, feels like you have a slight cold much of the time [mid to advanced cases]
4 ☐	Skin sensation, involuntary twitching of skin
3 ☐	Sleep for first two or three days on holiday
9 ☐	Sleep not very beneficial, or not beneficial at all, disturbed sleep.
2 ☐	Slightly sore skin on back and shoulders, possible rash on shins elbows or back
2 ☐	Slightly sore throat, dry or phlegm
6 ☐	Slow nail growth in general, rarely cut fingernails, lines or ridges on fingernails. [In advanced cases usually with impaired liver function or gallstones]
1 ☐	Sometimes feel slightly spaced out [more noticeable if you try eating wheat or drinking wine in the early stages of recovery]
3 ☐	Sore eyes stinging
10 ☐	Stomach-aches in general, often when hungry, you may feel like you have a ball just under your middle ribcage, sometimes the ache or pain may run through to your back [often in younger life as well as present day.]
3 ☐	Sweating excessively on hot days or when exercising.
2 ☐	Thick toenails. Often starts with fourth and fifth on right foot, or thick toenails in general [in advanced cases]
5 ☐	Tingling and numbness in fingers and toes [often when at rest with legs crossed or arms folded]
4 ☐	Tired but have problems sleeping, disturbed sleep.
10 ☐	Tiredness or exhaustion [in advanced stages maybe total debilitating tiredness, chronic fatigue or M.E]
1 ☐	Urine. Strong smelling acidic urine in your younger years.
10 ☐	Very gaseous and windy, with reflux [acid indigestion]
3 ☐	Waking up in the night feeling totally drained and exhausted [legs aching]
7 ☐	Yeast overgrowth, candida [good indication is yellowish white on top rear of tongue, most cases have this condition]

TOTAL SCORE: ☐

I compiled the List of symptoms above, after personal experience with food intolerance.
I had experienced all these symptoms in abundance by the age of 41.These symptoms were developing, one by one, throughout most of my early life.

Not all these symptoms may occur, It depends how advanced your food intolerance is, but people in the very advanced stages of food intolerance will recognise most, or all of these symptoms.

YOUR SCORE

0-10:   It is very unlikely that you are gaining food intolerance.

10-40:   If the ones you have ticked included some or most of the following, normal bowels, or constipation happening on occasion, stomach bloated occasionally, generally quite tired, gaseous and windy occasionally, indigestion occasionally. There is a reasonable possibility that you may have gained food intolerance. But you are in the early stages of food intolerance without further complications, or other symptoms.

40-60:   If the ones you have ticked included some or most of the following, bloated stomach, often normal bowels, sometimes constipated, occasionally loose, general tiredness, often gaseous and windy, acid reflux quite often, yeast overgrowth or Candida (whitish yellow growth on back of tongue), You have probably gained food intolerance to some degree and are advancing into more serious food intolerance.

60-90:   If the ones you have ticked included some or most of the following, bloated stomach, tiredness, gaseous and windy, acid reflux, constipation or loose bowels, or switching between the two, but sometimes normal, yeast overgrowth, Candida (whitish yellow growth on back of tongue), sensitive eyes, dry patches of skin, dead limbs when sleeping, tingling in fingers or toes, and sleep not very beneficial.

You are advancing into acute food intolerance and beginning to gain many of the symptoms associated with advancing intolerance.

90 –130:   If the ones you ticked included some or most of the following, feeling like you have a ball in your stomach, bloated stomach, switching between loose bowels and constipation, rarely normal bowel movements, tiredness, gaseous and windy, yeast overgrowth Candida (whitish yellow growth on back of tongue), light sensitive eyes, your eyes may also feel like they have grit in them, dry patches of skin, lines running length of fingernails, sleep not very beneficial, dead limbs when sleeping, bruised feeling in stomach or lower abdomen when tapped with fingers, bloated retentive appearance in face, and also your body, you might look and feel like the Michelin man, drained of energy on hot clammy days, slightly flu like feeling, aching back knees or shoulder, dry bottom lip and corners of mouth, tingling in fingers and toes. You are very advanced with chronic food intolerance and developing serious complications, you may even have been diagnosed with IBS or M.E

130 +:   You must have ticked all or virtually all the symptoms, then you will be extremely intolerant, to the foods I advise you not to eat. You will probably have loose bowels all the time, your digestive tract is probably in the emergency state, refer to pages 111 and 263 for an explanation of the emergency state.

It is possible that you could have developed other complications and been diagnosed with a problem such as, IBS, ulcerative colitis, diverticulitis, m.e (myalgic encephalitis, lupus, thyroid problems, iron deficient Anaemia, Crohn's disease, hypoglycaemia, Fibromyalgia, and others.

You will have to follow the recovery programme detailed in this book to the letter, to gain full recovery.

You will have to commit yourself fully to the advice given in this book, and will very quickly realise the consequences of stepping off the recovery programme and diet.

The points system above is a guide, but I usually find it to be a pretty accurate way to try and assess how far you have spiralled down the food intolerance chain.

However all these symptoms can be related to food intolerance, at some stage in the advancement of the condition.

It's extremely difficult to try and devise an infallible points guide, because the food intolerance phenomena can pause as many and varied symptoms, at different stages, in the advancement of food intolerance.

Some symptoms are a constant with very advanced food intolerance, such as bloating, tiredness, loose bowels, constipation, acid reflux with wind and gaseousness. Therefore these have high scores.

This can be quite a complicated subject because many diseases have the same symptoms; therefore you have to be very careful before deciding whether you have developed intolerance to food, or have an illness.

Diagnosing whether you are, or have developed intolerance to certain foods can be quite time consuming and complicated, so I am going to try and make it a little easier for you.

People who are very fit and healthy have no traceable pattern of any kind. Obviously they have been ill at some stage in their lives, but there is no connection between the events, and no common complaints, such as stomach ache. Unlike those of us who have gained or always had food intolerance.

It's like trying to piece together a 3,000,000 piece jigsaw, the more pieces of information you can gather, the more you can begin to see a picture of the whole problem. Then you can begin to recognise, and decide if this has been a life long, or life gained intolerance.

Over a period of time, as you grow older, it slowly begins to dawn on you, that there is something wrong, this is not normal. It can't just be my age. I can't have worn myself out through overwork or stress already, not at my age. Often "my age" can mean as young as 25 to 45 years old.

CLUES IN YOUNGER YEARS

People don't always show symptoms in their younger years, it depends at what age their digestive compromise begins to cause problems.

But just in case your liver was clogged as a baby, let's start at the beginning, when you were born. Ask your mother if you were a sickly baby especially if given milk, this is a very important indication of developing food intolerance later in life. Many intolerants report being very sickly when fed dried milk or dairy products as a baby; this is often accompanied by diarrhoea or loose bowels.

- If a baby develops diarrhoea when weaned onto wheat-based products then it is a good sign that they are susceptible to wheat. They are reacting in the main to the wheat gluten protein.

- Did you at school age often complain to mum of stomach-ache?

- Did you at school age have bouts of diarrhoea, or more often the case constipation?
- Constipation is often reported by the mothers of intolerants to have been a problem in their offspring when their son or daughter was a child of around 3 to 12 years old. Often these children subsequently go on to become intolerants; this is a very common occurrence with food intolerants.

- Were you often ill, off school with minor illnesses, colds fluey etc, were you often under the weather?

- Did you have glandular fever? This is another extremely common occurrence in intolerance sufferers.

- Did you have stomach problems?

- Did you have bad acne as a teenager, with some stomach discomfort?

- Were you light headed, easily faint?

- Did you have dark bags under your eyes?

- Were you very thin, and then begin to fill out in your late teenage years or late twenties?

- Did you have roseacea, (a very red and hot face, especially the cheeks, usually caused by sweet foods such as sugar, related to yeast overgrowth)

- Did car headlights or bright sunlight hurt your eyes, and make you squint?

The previous may seem vague questions on their own, but if we carry on building the picture through the teenage years and into your late teens and early twenties, we will get a more complete picture.

TEENS AND EARLY TWENTIES

Again some people don't show obvious signs of food intolerance until later in life.

As I said before, it depends at which point your digestive tract becomes compromised.

Anyway let's carry on building the picture. Did you still have stomach-aches? But could not attribute it to anything or maybe thought it was quite normal?

If playing football, squash, tennis, cricket, or any activities requiring physical exertion did you sweat excessively?

Could you not quite keep up with the other people, or seem to have to work extremely hard too keep up, and put it down to the drink at the weekend, or think, well I'm obviously just not built for this athletics thing.

Again, did, or do you have, loose bowels or constipation, or switching between the two.

• Were any broadband antibiotics taken for a length of time for any illnesses?

• Was irritable bowel diagnosed?

• Did your legs ache after a day at work?

• Did you need a sleep after coming home from work?

• Were your eyes red in the morning? No, no, not after a night on the drink, but regularly with slight stinging, and or a waxy or gritty feeling.

• Did you squint at bright sun light or car headlights?

• Was your urine very strong and acidic in your younger years? This is an indication of uric acid caused by too much protein in your diet. Refer to the kidney cleanse chapter and page 218.

MORE RECENTLY

• If you catch a cold have you found that they have become worse and worse over the years, and more intense, and harder to fight off?

• What is your recovery rate after a good night on the town, 1 day, 3 days, a week? This is a good indication of how fast your body detoxifies. By the way four days is extremely bad, good detoxifiers recover after a good nights sleep, and are affected very little the next day.

• If doing a physical job, do you find yourself tired at the end of the day, and having to sleep after coming home?

• Do you feel bloated and very full after meals, and think this is normal?

Think about the way you are or were then. This is not easy, because someone who is intolerant to food and always has been, maybe does not know what normal is. In the early years of your life, you don't tend to notice mild reactions, because your body is still growing. It's naturally able to cope with infiltration from foreign substances to a greater degree, without showing obvious reactions.

Some of the very early telltale signs of food intolerance, especially if you begin to gain your food intolerances after the age of 30 are, acid reflux, slight tingling in fingers and possibly toes, after having your legs crossed or arms folded.
• Bloating of stomach in men, and bloating of stomach, and possibly lower abdomen in women,
• Aching legs, especially knees.
• Aching shoulders.
• Stiff joints, and a slightly fluey feeling.
• Sleep not very beneficial.

As you become older your body slowly loses the ability to regenerate and then you go into the downward spiral of the symptom chain, and end up with the symptoms as listed on the first pages of this chapter.

I didn't realise some of these symptoms were actually symptoms in myself; until I took away the foods I was intolerant to. I now realise the devastating effect this can have on your body long term.

One of the main reasons why people don't realise they are intolerant to wheat, is that they eat it every day, and therefore they never or very rarely get away from it. Therefore your body has never had the chance to recover, even to the point where there is a small noticeable improvement in well-being.

Have you noticed that if you go on holiday abroad you feel better, and put it down to the sun and rest? Well this may not be the whole picture, because many foreign breads are not fortified as our home baked breads, and don't use flour containing high levels of gluten.

Most foreign bakers don't use the "Chorley Wood baking process" to accelerate the baking process, and therefore definitely do not have the same intense reaction as our home baked varieties. Plus when you are on holiday you don't tend to eat as many dairy products, which are very hard to break down.

On the plus side you tend to eat more fruit and salads when on holiday, this change in diet, and getting some sun, and more rest, can radically improve a food intolerants condition in as little as a week.

If you have become very food intolerant, you may find that you are bloated but still feel hungry, and are always raiding the kitchen at night to try and satisfy your hunger. Strangely, I found that you get a craving for the foods, which make you ill.

It's almost like you have become addicted to the foods that are making you intolerant. This is probably because you are not extracting and absorbing the elements in these foods, and your body is telling you subconsciously to eat more of these foods. It's leaving your hunger pangs turned on.

It's like a double-edged sword where sometimes you may feel full, but are still hungry. This may sound silly and a contradiction in terms, but those of you in the advanced stages of intolerance will know exactly what I mean.

THE MID LIFE REPRIEVE

I often find the same life-long pattern in people with wheat, dairy intolerance, although I have found quite a few cases of sufferers who show very little sign of intolerance in their teenage and middle years. Although they may have the traceable pattern in their younger years, mainly as a baby, when they were sick if fed powdered or cows milk.

They only begin to develop the many food intolerance symptoms, as listed on pages 18 to 21 in their later years, usually aged 35 to 50 or even 60. The digestive system in these people seems to control the food intolerance, other than say acid reflux, and slight bloating, in their middle years. They then become food intolerant very quickly, often within a couple of years.

If you fall into this group of people, you will find that you could rapidly develop many of the symptoms in as little as one year, usually in your late thirties or early forties.

Often I can find something that has tipped them over the edge into advanced intolerance, such as a minor operation, an illness, stress, taking antibiotics, or taking medications like very strong antacids, or acid suppressants (protein pump inhibitors), often for the aforementioned acid reflux.

A bad fall, or exercise such as squat thrusts, or lifting weights up and down with your legs can dislodge gallstones, moving them into a position where they partially block your common bile duct. This can make your system trip into food intolerance within a few weeks, or even days.

Some people are tipped over the edge when they stop smoking," what and how I hear you cry!" If you stop smoking you often eat more food, and often more of the wrong food. Remember you have or are losing the ability to break down some foods, such as wheat and dairy products, so if you eat more of these foods it is often enough to trip the digestive tract into the more advanced reactive states, such as loose bowels, or even the emergency state as described on pages 111-263.

Any of the aforementioned can be responsible for a rapid decline in digestive function. Often your digestive system has just been coping until the LAST STRAW BREAKS THE CAMELS BACK, This can overwhelm your digestive system, and other organs, making you rapidly begin to fall into the mire of food intolerance, losing your ability to break down and absorb many of the elements in the foods we all eat on a daily basis.

PARENTS, BROTHERS AND SISTERS, SONS AND DAUGHTERS

An extremely good indication of food intolerance, is to look at the health of your parents, and other members of your family.

If you are a definite food intolerant then one, or other, of your parents is definitely, absolutely, without doubt, in every case, a food intolerant to one degree or another. I have yet to find a food intolerant who has not got a food intolerant parent
It is quite possible that both of your parents are intolerants, this is often the case.
It's vital to look at your parents and see if you can work out which one of or even both them, have had or have any obvious symptoms, such as the aforementioned stomach problems.

Are or were they always tired in their later years and complaining of stomach-ache? Only you can reach a rational conclusion on this subject. Quiz them about some of the symptoms of intolerance. You will have some knowledge of the subject by the time you have reached the stage of getting ill, and very desperate, and turning to this book for help.

Take note of brothers or sisters, especially if there are more than 2 siblings, have any of them been diagnosed with irritable bowel, do they get stomach-aches etc, etc. I say this because it's unusual to say the least, not to find at least one other sibling of your family who has not gained, or always had, food intolerance.

There is a definite link between parent and child with food intolerance, and you can almost always see an obvious, staring you in the face, common symptoms criteria, between parent and child.

If you are a parent, and a food intolerant, you must look at your own children; do they show any obvious signs of food intolerance, rashes, bloating, stomach-ache on a regular basis, spots, inability to put on weight, very thin, weary, tired etc? If you have say four children and you are definitely a food intolerant, then there is an overwhelming, in fact almost certain probability that one of your offspring is also food intolerant.

If there are signs of food intolerance, any one of them could be intolerant. There is no rule of thumb here, it depends on what they have inherited, but if both parents are intolerant then you can be quite sure the offspring will be.

I have three daughters, Charlotte, Kirsty and Sophie. If they were fed a high wheat diet they began to show signs of food intolerance, so we kept them on a low wheat and dairy products diet.

I was sure by Charlotte's reactions to wheat and dairy products that she had gallstones. So when she was 15 years old she flushed out her gallbladder and liver, and lo and behold she flushed out hundreds of gallstones, and lots of chaff, yes at 15 years old.

Now she can tolerate small amounts of wheat, eats very little sugar and dairy, and reports that she feels far less tired and has more energy, since the flushes her stomach aches have totally gone.

But more interestingly my other 2 daughters, Kirsty and Sophie, are identical twins, you couldn't tell them apart when they were young, unless they were stood together. However by the time they were 8, Kirsty had become slightly bloated and Sophie was much thinner and more delicate. You could easily tell them apart.

I was amazed to find that after vastly reducing their wheat intake and dramatically reducing their dairy and sugar intake, kirsty lost her bloated appearance and Sophie began to fill out more. By the time they were 12 they were almost identical again.

This only serves to confirm and reinforce my views and convictions that wheat has a detrimental effect on the digestive tract in young children, if they are susceptible.

The most worrying observation is that the children of intolerants often appear to be more intolerant than their parents; It's as though the ability of their digestive tract is being eroded with each generation, although it is far to early for me to come to any absolute conclusion on this observation, it may be that our modern diet is just becoming more and more laden with wheat, dairy, and sugar based products, and that there are more additives, and preservatives affecting us throughout our lives.

DIARY OF FOODS AND REACTION CHART

If at the end of this you may think you have become a food intolerant, you can monitor what you eat. Keeping a record of what you eat, and your reactions to the foods you have eaten, in a diary.

In my case I devised the charts and records on the next four pages, to record the reactions to what I ate, and then keep a record of what I ate, visits to the toilet, and any other reactions in my diary.

Although I have to say, I very much doubt you will want to go to these lengths, because this is a very tedious undertaking. The list of foods you cannot eat on page 14 (the chart you can cut out as a reference) or refer to the same list on pages 42 to 45 generally covers most food intolerants. If this list is adhered to it should stabilise your digestive tract, saving you the tedium of making lists and keeping charts and diaries as I did.

I devised this chart, which I found invaluable. As you can see by the chart a vast amount of information can be gathered, and by far the greatest task is to analyse it.

The vast amount of information it produced enabled me to pin down the intolerant foods, and even the reactions of combinations of foods.

If some types of food are eaten with the foods you are intolerant to, they will have the effect of moderating the extreme reaction of the intolerant food, and confusing the issue. This is the main reason why it's so difficult to arrive at a definite list of foods that you may have become intolerant to.

Over the page is the key to the symbols etc, in relation to the reactions chart on the next page.

The letter S
means that I felt about average, about the same as I would on an average day whilst in the depths of my food intolerance.

The up arrow in blue ↑
This means I felt better and the number indicates by how much on a scale of 1-8.
1 being a slight improvement and 8 being a vast improvement.

The down arrow in red ↓
This means I felt worse and the number indicates by how much on a scale of 1 –8.
1 being slightly worse, and 8 being very bad.

The letter T
This means a visit to the Toilet, and I kept a record in my diary of the type of stools that had formed.

The spot sign ●
This means I ate something and kept a record of it in my diary.

As you can see in an instant on the chart on the next page, the 15, 16, and 17th June were better days, and a look in the diary on pages 30-33 gives some clues, this was the turning point, and after this I quickly began to pin down all the offending foods, and felt much better in little time.

TIME OF DAY	07.30	08.00	08.30	09.00	09.30	10.00	10.30	11.00	11.30	12.00	12.30
MONDAY 12 JUNE	● ↓ 1	↓ 6	↓ T 6	↓ 6	↓ T 6	● S	S	S	S	S	● T S
TUESDAY 13 JUNE	● S	↓ T 6	↓ 8	↓ 8	↓ T 6	● ↓ 4	↓ 4	↓ 4	↓ T 4	↓ 2	● S
WEDNESDAY 14 JUNE	● ↓ 2	↓ 3	↓ 3	↓ T 3	↓ 3	● ↓ 3	↓ 4	↓ 4	↓ 4	↓ 3	● ↓ 4
THURSDAY 15 JUNE	● S	S	S	T S	S	● S	S	↑ 2	↑ 3	↑ 4	● ↑ T 4
FRIDAY 16 JUNE	● ↓ 2	S	S	S	↑ 2	● ↑ 4	↑ 6	↑ 6	↑ 6	↑ T 6	● ↑ 7
SATURDAY 17 JUNE	● T S	S	S	S	S	↑ 4	↑ 6	↑ 8	↑ 8	↑ 8	↑ 8
SUNDAY 18 JUNE	● ↓ 8	↓ T 8	↓ 8	↓ 8	↓ T 8	● ↓ 8	↓ 8	● ↓ 8	↓ T 8	↓ 8	● ↓ 8

13.00	13.30	14.00	14.30	15.00	15.30	16.00	16.30	17.00	17.30	18.00	19.00	20.00	21.00	22.00
S	↓6	↓7	↓8	•↓8	↓8	↓8	↓7	↓4	↓2	•↓2	↓2	↓4	↓4	•↓3
S	↑T6	↑2	↑3	•↑3	↑3	↑3	↑3	↑4	↑4	•↑4	S	↓2	↓4	•↓T7
↓5	↓6	↓8	↓8	•↓8	↓8	↓8	↓8	↓7	↓T6	•↓6	↓T7	↓8	↓8	•↓6
↑4	↑2	↑4	↑4	•↑4	↑4	↑5	↑5	↑5	↑5	•↑5	↑2	T S	•↓1	↓2
↑7	↑7	↑7	↑7	•↑7	↑8	↑8	↑8	↑8	↑8	•↑8	↑8	↑T8	•↑8	↑8
•↑8	↑	S	↓2	↓4	↓5	↓5	S	T S	↑1	•↑1	↑2	↑2	S	•↓T2
↓8	↓7	↓6	•↓5	↓4	↓3	↓2	•S	T S	S	•S	S	S	•↓2	↓6

MEAL	BREAKFAST	LUNCH
MONDAY **12 JUNE**	Corn Flakes, 4 Slices Toast, Cup Of Tea, *10.00: T Pungent, Bulky* Bag Crisps Cup Tea	Steak Pie, Chips And Gravy a Slice Of Bread, Strawberry Yoghurt, Can Of Coke. Tea *T Pungent, Bulky*
TUESDAY **13 JUNE**	Egg, bacon, 2 fried bread, cup of tea, orange juice *8.30 and 9.30 T very loose,* *light coloured* 10.00 am, yoghurt, cup tea	4 Salmon sandwiches Strawberry yoghurt Biscuit coffee *11.30 T loose*
WEDNESDAY **14 JUNE**	Cornflakes, 2 slices toast Cup of tea Orange juice *T pungent v loose* 10.00 2 cheese sandwich, cup tea	4 cheese sandwiches Yoghurt, Bag crisps 4 digestive Biscuits Cup coffee Can coke
THURSDAY **15 JUNE**	Corn flakes Egg bacon tomato Orange juice Cup tea *T loose* 10.00 yoghurt cup tea	Tin beans Banana, Apple 4 digestive biscuits Cup tea *T loose still recognise foods*
FRIDAY **16 JUNE**	Corn flakes Egg bacon tomato Orange juice Cup tea 10.00 yoghurt, cup tea	Cheese and biscuits Banana Pear Cup tea *T loose*
SATURDAY **17 JUNE**	Corn flakes, Egg bacon tomato, Orange, Cup tea 10.00 Cup tea *T loose*	Steak pie chips peas and gravy Can coke *T firmer, sl darker*

DINNER	SUPPER
Mashed potatoes, fish fingers, fruit salad and custard. 2 slices bread. Tea *15.00 T firmer*	Cup tea Apple, 2 salmon sandwiches. Went to bed 10.30
Cornish pasty Potatoes, peas, gravy Pears and cream 2 slices bread, tea *15.00 T firmer*	Corn flakes Ham sandwich Cheese sandwich Cup tea Cup milk *T firmer*
Cheese and onion pie, chips, peas, gravy. 1 slice bread Pears and custard, 2 digestive biscuits, cup tea *15.00 T very loose*	Corn flakes 4 digestive biscuits Banana Cup tea *T very loose*
Steak and kid pie Potatoes, carrots Gravy, Rice pudding *Cup tea and pear at 15.00*	Cup tea Corn flakes 2 biscuits with cheese Pot noodle *T firmer, pungent*
Cheese and ham salad Peaches and custard Cup tea Cup tea and apple at 15.00	Cup tea 6 biscuits with cheese Packet crisps Banana *T Firmer, sl darker*
Fish , potatoes cauliflower, and cheese sauce Peaches in jelly and cream, Cup tea	6 pints lager Fish chips *T loose*

This meal cycle continued on a six-day basis from Sunday 18 June onwards.

NOTES IN DIARY

Mon 12th June
- Woke up in night with dead arms and legs again
- Felt bloated
- Windy all afternoon
- Slightly better at night
- Still pain in stomach, and occasionally lower down.
- Very tired, bed 10.00

Tue 13th June
- Eyes full of wax
- Tingling in fingers and feet
- Felt bloated in morning
- Slightly better in afternoon
- Stomach- ache tonight

Wed 14th June
- Woke up last night
- Hard to sleep, although very tired
- Drained
- Aching legs and exhausted
- Stomach-ache, bad after lunch
- Sat down for 10 minutes
- Pains in lower stomach area
- Slight improvement tonight
- Very tired
- Had think, leave out bread tomorrow.

Thur 15th June
- Average this morning
- Felt slightly better in morning
- Definitely better in afternoon
- Not as windy
- Less stomach-ache
- Gone worse again tonight
- Could be bread, yeast

Fri 16th June
- Still tingling in toes and fingers
- Slightly "off" this morning
- Definitely less bloated
- Stomach more settled especially bowels

- Better in morning and this afternoon
- Starving hungry tonight
- Very tired

Sat 17th June
- Woke in night aching
- Definitely better in stomach
- Less bloated in morning, worse in afternoon.
- Must be bread or something in it, but none at lunch and had reaction.
- About same tonight.

One day of this information on its own, does not say a lot, but if you analysed a month's statistics very carefully, you learn to use the system and glean information from it.

For instance, some foods like milk seem to have a two to three hour reaction time, and a four-day recovery time.

But wine reacts in less than 20 minutes, and has a about a twelve hour recovery time, this reaction will be more acute if you have yeast or bacterial overgrowth, Candida.

As I said before, it's unlikely that you would use this chart, as it is too time consuming for most people, just use the lists in this book. These food lists cover most food intolerants, and should enable recovery to take place.

There are many ways to determine intolerance to food; I will just run through a few.

You could try leaving out foods and see if there is a good or bad reaction; this is called an elimination diet. You start by eating virtually nothing but greens and then slowly re introducing foods into your diet, and monitor your reaction. Although in my experience this is not always the best method, because some foods don't necessarily show a reaction if eaten on their own, but may do so if combined with other foods, such as eating cheese with pasta, cheese on its own has very little reaction and small quantities of pasta have very little reaction, but combine the two and quite a severe reaction will be the result.

Other foods if combined, may often cancel out any reaction, for instance if you ate tuna with a slice of bread, the reaction to the gluten is very much reduced, the tuna helps to neutralise the effects of the gluten in the bread.

You may go for an allergy test, but again it doesn't always unearth all your intolerances, and often the one it doesn't unearth is wheat intolerance, plus many of the findings of these allergy tests often give conflicting information, take gluten for instance, if you show a reaction to wheat gluten then surely you should show a reaction to the gluten in oats, as they are one and the same, so someone could be told to eat oats but not wheat, this would not stabilise their condition.

This test is usually done by what is known as a wheatstone bridge, where a small current is passed through a hand held probe, then varying foods and elements are inserted in the machine and this indicates a reaction or not.

Another method of testing for intolerance is the pulse method, where you go on an elimination diet and then take your pulse every few minutes over the period of an hour, after introducing different foods. If your pulse rate is elevated, it is supposed to indicate intolerance of the food you have just ingested.

This is not easy for the inexperienced in this method, and I have to say, not very accurate.

None of these tests are informative enough. They don't tell you that if you take away the wheat and other foods, then clean out the liver and clean the kidneys; the intolerances go away after some time.

I went for 7 weeks using the chart method I had devised, and could not quite trace a definite pattern. I was eliminating all sorts from the sandwiches I took to work, but stupid me had not thought about the obvious, the bread.

The reason I did not think about the bread was the fact that I had 2 biopsies for celiac disease, but after the first biopsy, which is were I was when doing these experiments, I was told that I was not a celiac, so I assumed I was not intolerant to bread, or more to the point, gluten.

But after a while it began to dawn on me that the bread was definitely causing a problem,
It definitely was not the yeast in the bread, I had tried raw yeast with little effect, and it was not the other elements in the bread as my doctor had suggested may be the case, I had tried many of the other elements in the bread, such as Thiamine, Niacin, Riboflavin, calcium, iron, in large doses, with little or no effect, there was only one obvious left, the gluten. So I sourced some high gluten content flour (72% extraction) and ate quite a quantity of it, within 2 hours I felt like death was imminent, my stomach exploded and turned into a witches cauldron of gas, cramping, bloating, and unbelievable discomfort, this reaction took about six hours to subside and left me with very loose bowels for three days after, and sure enough once I left out the bread or to be more precise the Gluten, which was now beyond doubt affecting me, everything else began to fall into place.

After this enlightening event and many more dramatic experiments, I eventually arrived at the list of foods you cannot eat, if your digestive system has degraded to the point that mine had.

The most amazing reaction was the 3 inches I lost off my waist, in the first two weeks after I eliminated the wheat from my diet. Yes I know that sounds amazing! I now know this was due to the inflammation subsiding within my stomach, and bowel.

INTENSE REACTION

Inevitably if you have all the symptoms on pages 18 to 21, I can tell you that you are extremely intolerant, and your first and trigger intolerance is wheat. Even a very small ingestion will affect you, even one biscuit.

If you swept up the crumbs after making sandwiches and ingested them, it would affect you noticeably, especially if you have not ingested any wheat products for a week or so in the early stages and then eaten some.

The dairy intolerance runs alongside the wheat intolerance, and will only disappear after a series of gallbladder and liver flushes, the flushes must only be completed after a period on this diet. Dairy products don't appear to have as devastating an affect on the digestive system; there are two main reasons why you react to dairy products.

1 The first is that dairy products are hard to break down, mainly due to being pasteurised, killing all the natural bacteria in the milk, leaving your digestive tract to do all the work in breaking it down. Dairy products will tend to wash through your digestive tract undigested; this will make you tired and possibly loose bowelled.

2 The other reason is the lactose (milk sugar) in dairy products, will feed your yeast overgrowth, further upsetting gut flora.

Many people take away just the dairy products and feel much better, but they are still not right, and don't realise that they will also be intolerant to wheat.

They don't realise they are only taking away a consequence of wheat intolerance, and digestive malfunction, and not the causal factor of their dairy intolerance, which is the inability to break down gluten in wheat.

All these intolerances are induced by a clogged liver, decreased pancreatic function and sluggish kidneys.

OTHER OBSERVED SYMPTOMS

When I first started analysing my symptoms I found maybe 12 diseases or conditions I could have had, but after detailed experimenting and using the symptoms chart, I managed to pin down the causal factor to wheat, or some element in flour.

Food intolerance is a most illusive condition. Many diseases, illnesses, or conditions can be read into the varying symptoms that many food intolerants present with.
If you just take the symptoms on the surface, you could very easily misdiagnose the problem, and relate them to traditionally, singular, separately treated conditions. Conventional medicine has, in the past, treated conditions such as, acid reflux, pancreatitis, diverticulitis, ulcerative colitis or I.B.S. separately, with drugs of one kind or another. I now realise that these common conditions should be treated under the same umbrella, because they have the same causal factor, as you will understand after reading this book.

After all the experimenting on myself, and observation of hundreds of other people with the same food intolerances, I have found intolerance to wheat, to be the best mimic of other diseases or conditions you will ever find.

It can take on many guises, and pose as other conditions. This can often make it very hard to diagnose, and often the only true test is to completely eliminate wheat from the diet.

Initially we thought I may have celiac disease (a reaction to the gluten protein element in wheat) but after having blood tests and two biopsies this proved not to be the case, although the medical profession agreed to treat me as a celiac, because the second biopsy was deemed to be borderline.

It goes deeper than the obvious conditions a doctor would read into your symptoms, on a short visit to the surgery.

For instance I had many symptoms; yeast overgrowth, arthritic symptoms, osteoarthyrsis, (aching and swelling joints), irritable bowel syndrome (I.B.S) dermatitis herpetiformis (red spots on dry skin), chronic fatigue ME, (myalgic encephalitis) hypoglycaemia (low blood sugar level), and all the symptoms in the list on pages 18 to 21.

I also had both gallstone, and pancreatic symptoms.

Regarding the gallbladder symptoms. I had pain in the front lower rib cage and running through to my back, and in the right front lower rib cage, running around my right hand side, into and under my right hand shoulder blade. The pancreatic symptoms were, pain under my lower middle ribcage, running through and out of the middle of my back. With these pancreas and gall bladder symptoms, you would expect to feel quite nauseous on a regular basis, but I did not have very much nausea at all.

I now know for certain that the gained food intolerance was causing respiratory problems, because I now have much more lung capacity than when I was in the depths of intolerance.

Cystic fibrosis type symptoms albeit relatively mild were there. In the case of my cystic fibrosis type symptoms, my lungs used to gurgle when taking my first breath after sleep, and I found I very easily got short of breath and patently did not appear to produce enough enzymes, because taking substitute enzymes helped a great deal. This was also a good indication that my pancreas was not functioning very efficiently, your pancreas produces enzymes, these help to break down starches, proteins, and fats in your digestive tract.

I have found some cases, where people have been found to have iron deficient anaemia after giving blood. We have found at a later date that they are definitely intolerant to wheat and dairy products, the anaemia goes away as they clean their liver and kidneys, and advance in recovery.

It's unlikely that you will have all the previously mentioned symptoms, unless you have long established food intolerance, or chronic fatigue as I had.
If you do have all the symptoms in the list on pages 18 to 21, then there is a strong possibility that you also have gallstones, and a series of gallbladder and liver flushes is essential, as detailed in the gallbladder flush chapter.

Even if you only have a few of these symptoms it has to be well worth doing a gall bladder flush, because this will flush out any chaff in the liver, even if gall stones are not present, it can only improve your digestive tracts ability to produce more bile and enzymes, and therefore you will break down and more importantly absorb what you eat much better.

At one time I was so intolerant to foods that many things upset my digestive tract. This made it quite difficult to arrive at the true food intolerance list.
For instance if I ate certain foods such as carrots and sweet corn, they came out in my stools almost as recognisable as when they were ingested.

I was convinced I was not producing enough enzymes or bile, so I asked my doctor for a faecal test and pancreatic tests. They did this after about 4 months, but by this time I had recovered quite markedly.

To my amazement all the test results came back as normal, but I still patently was not breaking down or absorbing foods properly. All I can say is, you must have to be seriously ill before the test parameters recognise or define a problem.

So after being on the wheat/dairy exemption diet for about 12months, virtually all of the symptoms went away. All I was left with was the definite gallbladder-type symptoms, albeit mild symptoms. These symptoms were being masked by the bloating and other related problems in the early days of recovery.

So, I approached my doctor with a view to having a gallbladder scan or other tests, but he seemed reluctant. But after a while he relented, and I had an ultrasound scan of my gallbladder and liver, and the doctor said my gallbladder looked a little unusual, but he was sure there were no gallstones present and everything looked ok.

I have to say I was a little surprised, so I decided to try and find a gallstone, or gall bladder cure myself.

After sifting through and trying many so-called cures, my sister Janet stumbled across a gall bladder flush.

I have to say that this was one of the only ones I looked at, that I thought might just work, because it made sense. So I tried it, and to my amazement passed over 2400 gallstones, although I had to do 26 flushes, 120 were as big as a bean, and approximately 1400 the size of a small pea, and hundreds of others too soft and small to collect, and lots and lots of chaff in the latter flushes.

Then I realised I still had some slight discomfort in my kidney area, and so I cleaned out my kidneys using the beetroot juice and later on using the herbal cleanse. This definitely eliminated the discomfort in my kidney area, and I improved immensely after these treatments.

It looked like I had finally found the last problems in curing my condition. My symptoms and food intolerances slowly went away, but it took two years or so for them to die down fully.

You may say that was what was wrong with me all along, but I now know through my life history, and the reactions and symptoms of others, that the gallstones and clogged liver are as a consequence of poor diet over a lifetime, leading to the inability to break down food and consequently food intolerances.

The causal factors are to my understanding, the over indulgence over a lifetime in highly processed, high gluten protein wheat, pasteurised dairy products, and to a large degree processed sugar.

YEAST OVERGROWTH

Almost invariably I can tell you that if you have some of the symptoms listed on pages 164, you will have yeast overgrowth to one degree or another. The dietary regime will have to be followed to eradicate it, along with a series of gallbladder and liver flushes, and the kidney cleanses. Refer to the yeast overgrowth chapter on page 171, for the foods you will have to avoid, to help eradicate yeast overgrowth.

HELICOBACTER PYLORI

Another problem you may have is a bacterium, which many of the population have, called Helicobacter Pylori. This often does not affect fit and healthy people, they do not present with any symptoms, but in the case of food intolerance it can cause stomach-aches, ulcers, and inflammation, and prevent a recovery.

It is very easy to discover whether or not you have Helicobacter Pylori, a simple blood test at your doctors will identify whether you have the bacterium or not.

More information on Helicobacter Pylori can be found on page 162.

FOODS THAT CANNOT BE EATEN

People who are intolerant to wheat are almost invariably intolerant to dairy products, anyone who knows they are intolerant to dairy products are also intolerant to wheat although they often don't realise this.

If the wheat products are taken away along with the dairy products they improve markedly.

Their first intolerance is wheat, mainly bread flour, and not solely the dairy products as many people often think, the reasons for this are explained in the, "What happens to the digestive tract" chapter, on pages 100-112.

Below is a list in alphabetical order of the foods you cannot eat, there is also the same list of "foods that cannot be eaten" on page 14, which can be cut from the book, and pinned to the kitchen wall as a quick reference.

You must start by not eating any of the foods listed in this chapter for the first TWO WEEKS.

You must stay away from any of the foods listed under WHEAT PRODUCTS, DAIRY PRODUCTS and SOYA PRODUCTS / TOFU until full recovery, or at least until most of the gallbladder and liver flushes required, have been completed.

After two weeks try introducing some of foods listed under OTHER INTOLERANCE FOODS, on page 45, (also on the cut out list of "foods that cannot be eaten") on page 14.

Try them one by one, if they react with you then you are very intolerant, and you must remove them from your diet again, beware of these foods in early recovery.

Wheat Products

• Barley

• Biscuits [most kinds contain wheat]

• Bran and bran related cereals

• Breakfast cereals [some are malt flavoured, and some are wheat or bran, which will react with you, also contain amounts of phytic acid, and gluten]

• Bulgar [dried wheat]

• Cheese [some cheeses, especially yellow ones and mouldy ones may contain an element of wheat]

• Couscous [made from wheat]

• Curry mixes [may contain wheat flour]

- Dried meals [may contain wheat flour]

- Durum [a type of wheat]

- Flour [wholemeal, granary, brown, bread]

- Ginger beer [may contain wheat colouring]

- Gravy mixes [contain flour]

- Ice cream [some contain wheat starch]

- Lager, beer, stout [they potentially contain residues of wheat]

- Lemonade [may contain wheat based colourings]

- Macaroni

- Mustard powder [may contain wheat]

- Oats [similar gluten to wheat, may not affect all with this condition, also contains phytic acid]

- Packet and tinned products [read labels all could have wheat starch or flour in them]

- Pasta [made from wheat]

- Peanuts [beware some salted peanuts, they may contain wheat starch]

- Pills [they may be bound with a wheat-based product]

- Rice paper [some use wheat flour]

- Rye [contains gluten similar to wheat]

- Salad cream [contains vinegar and therefore possible wheat]

- Sausages [contain flour]

- Sauces [may contain wheat starch]

- Semolina [made from wheat]

- Soy sauce [fermented in wheat flower]

- Spaghetti [made from wheat]

- Spelt [similar protein]

- Stock cubes and gravy cubes [may contain wheat]

- Starch [vegetable starch in processed or tinned food, this may be wheat starch]

- Toffees [some are dusted with wheat or have wheat starch]

- Tomato sauce [contains vinegar and therefore possible wheat]

- Triticale

- Vinegar [contains wheat]

- Vitamin E pills [usually made from wheat] source non-wheat derived vitamin E.

- Wheat germ

In virtually all cases if you are intolerant to wheat products you will be intolerant to dairy products, until the digestive system has recovered, this may take about 20 to 24 months, the reasons for this are covered in the, "what happens to the digestive tract" chapter.

Dairy Products:

- Biscuits

- Butter

- Cakes [many contain dairy products, obviously they contain wheat too]

- Cheese

- Chocolate

- Creams

- Ice cream

- Margarine

- Milk

- Some confectionary

- Yoghurt (plain live or bio yoghurt is all right and should be eaten, as detailed in the recovery programme, if you are an extreme intolerant and cannot even cope with the live yoghurt, then take pre and pro biotics, every day instead, as prescribed by your health shop, also detailed in the recovery programme)

Soya Products / Tofu:
Read all labels on products and avoid if Soya is present, people are often intolerant to Soya until some gallbladder and liver flushes have been completed. (Meat could be Soya substitute meat)

Other Intolerance Foods:
Other products that people often report react with them, when they are intolerant to wheat and dairy products, are the ones listed below, if you are intolerant to any of these products you must be very food intolerant, and therefore you will certainly require a series of gallbladder and liver flushes.

These products certainly affected me in the depths of my food intolerance, although the intolerance to these will go away once you have recovered, or as you advance in your recovery.

Try these other intolerance food products after two weeks, and gauge your reaction, most people can usually cope with most of the following foods even in early recovery.

Eggs
Be wary, sometimes people are intolerant in very early recovery.
Try them after the first two weeks and gauge your reaction.

Lemons, Limes
Very acidic, irritates stomach in early recovery, and often until some gallbladder and liver flushes have been completed.

Melons
This seems to be quite a common one in early recovery.

Orange
Juices, Still orange, Fresh orange
People are always intolerant to oranges until later in recovery, or at least until a few gallbladder and liver flushes have been completed.

Sesame Seeds
In extreme intolerance cases sesame seeds will react with you.

Stearic Acid
Beware of in tablets, if it's in a concentrated form it may react with you.

Tomatoes
In rare cases tomatoes may give you acid reflux in early recovery, and until some gallbladder and liver flushes have been done.

Cucumber
In very rare cases cucumber may react with you.

NB all the foods in the following list may be eaten in normal quantities after full recovery.

FOODS THAT CAN BE EATEN

Before you attempt this diet I would advise you to go shopping and stock your kitchen with the foods you can eat, otherwise you will find it very difficult to stick to the diet.

Do not be put off embarking on this diet just because you think it is very limited, and may be difficult to stick to, it is a change in your approach to the food you eat, and once you have begun this diet you will see a dramatic change in your well being, in as little as one or two weeks, this will encourage you to continue with the recovery programme.

So many people say to me that the one thing that keeps them on the diet is the fact that if they step off it they feel so ill, and they quickly revert to many of the symptoms listed in this book.

As I have said before in this book be careful when purchasing your food, you can buy many gluten and dairy free products, often in the "free from" section in supermarkets, but many of these contain elements which may upset your digestive tract, so be wary of them, they may contain sugar, wheat starch, caffeine or even other ingredients, not necessarily included in the ingredients list, these may also react with you.

Don't assume because they are wheat, gluten or dairy free that they will be all right for you to eat. I have also found that many gluten free breads react with most food intolerants, you may try these breads, but I would advise you not to eat them in early recovery.

 # All the foods on the list carrying this symbol, are related to yeast overgrowth.

This is a difficult one. I have left this symbol off some potentially sweet fruits, because they contain helpful enzymes and other elements, which help your digestive tract to break them down.

I would advise you to stay off the foods showing the # symbol for the first two months or so, if yeast overgrowth is present which it usually is, then you would definitely be better staying off them for the first two months. Once the yeast overgrowth is under control you will be able to start having small servings of these foods, this is usually after a number of gallbladder and liver flushes.

Jams are definitely out if yeast overgrowth is present because of their sugary content.

Some of the others not showing this symbol are potentially sugary, and encourage yeast overgrowth, but I have found that fruit such as Pineapple and grapefruit aid digestion, and if they are taken in small quantities in their own juice, and not in syrup, are more beneficial than detrimental, although if you are extremely intolerant you may even react to the pineapple or grapefruit, try them and gauge your reaction to them.

Fruits like apples, bananas, pears are all right, although the pears could have a very slight adverse reaction if very ripe.

Avocado pear is an excellent all round food, but will affect you in the early stages of recovery, if eaten in large amounts, this is due to its high fat content, and partly the amount of vit E it contains, potentially it is very difficult to break down, and the high vit E content may detoxify you too quickly.
If you have very bad yeast overgrowth, then there is every likely-hood that you have gallstones, or at the very least an impaired or clogged liver, and a series of gallbladder and liver flushes is recommended.

? All these products are oily or fatty and if you are in the advanced stages of intolerance you will not be able to cope with large servings of these foods.

I realised after much experimentation on myself, and other food intolerants, that our digestive tracts could not break down oily or fatty products in large amounts, in the early stages of recovery, especially if the people I experimented with were in the advanced stages of food intolerance, with permanent loose bowels (the emergency state).

In the advanced stages of intolerance, you will not be producing enough bile, and enzymes, to cope with large amounts of oils or fats, if you still cannot cope with large servings of oils and fats, even after 2 months on the recovery diet, it is almost certain that you will have many gallstones, and a series of gall bladder and liver flushes is a must do to attain recovery.

Wallchart List
The list on the next page is in alphabetical order, making it easy to trace foods your not sure whether you can eat or not at a glance.

There is also a list of "foods that can be eaten" on page 15, you can cut this out and pin it to the kitchen wall, and see at a glance what you can eat.

The symbols ? and # are to help to identify oily foods which are difficult for you to break down, and sugary foods which may feed your yeast overgrowth.

Remember after full recovery you can eat all of the foods in the following list, in any quantity you like.

WALLCHART

\# foods relating to yeast overgrowth (candida albicans) (eat small amounts of these, and only after the first two months)
? Oily and fatty foods, difficult to break down. (eat small amounts of these)

A
Almonds
Apples
Apricots #
Artichoke
Asparagus
Aubergine
Avocado pear
(small amm at first)

B
Bacon-?
Bamboo shoots
Bananas
Bean sprouts
Beans kidney
Beans runner
Beef, minced, corned-?
Beetroot
Bilberries #
Blackberries #
Blackcurrants #
Bloater fish
Blueberries #
Brawn-?
Broccoli
Brussels sprouts
Buckwheat flour

C
Cabbage
Carrots
Cashew nuts
Cauliflower
Caviar
Celeriac
Celery
Cherries #
Chestnuts

Chicken (without skin)
Chickpeas
Chicory
Cockles
Coconut
Codfish
Corn flour
Corn on the cob
Corn
Corned beef-?
Courgettes
Crab
Cranberries
Crayfish
Cress
Crisps (plain rarely as a treat)
Cucumber (be wary of)
Currants #

D
Dates #
Dripping-?
Duck

E
Eels
Eggs(be wary of in early recovery))
Endive

F
Fennel
Figs #
Flax seed
Fruit (not oranges) #
Fruit salad (no oranges) #

G
Gammon ham (boiled)
Garlic

(small amounts at first)
Gherkins
Ginger
Goose
Gooseberries #
Grapefruit (in own juice)
small ammounts
Grapes #
Greengage
Grouse

H
Haddock
Hake
Halibut
Ham-?
Hare-?
Hazelnuts
Heart-?
Herring-?
Honey #

J
Jams #

K
Kale
Ketchup #
Kidney beans
Kidney-?
Kippers-?
Kiwi Fruit #

L
Lamb-?
Leek
Lemon (small ammounts)
Lemonade #
Lentils
Lettuce

Limes (small ammounts)
Liver-?
Lobster
Loganberries #
Luncheon meat-?
M
Mackerel-?
Maize
Mango
Marrow
Mayonnaise-?
Mint
Mung beans
Mushrooms #
Mussels
Mutton-?

O
Oil, Vegetable, Olive etc-?
Okra
Olives-?
Onion (small amounts at first)
Oranges (beware of)
Oysters

P
Palm Hearts
Papaya
Parsley
Parsnips
Partridge
Peach #
Peanuts
(beware some brands contain wheat)
Pears
Peas
Pepper
Peppermint (not toffee mints)
Pheasant

Pilchards-?
Pine nuts
Pineapples (in own juice) small amounts
Plaice
Plums #
Pomegranate
Pork-?
Potatoes
Prawns
Prunes #
Phsyllum seeds
Pumpernickel
Pumpkin
Pumpkin seeds

R
Rabbit-?
Radish
Raisins #
Raspberries #
Redcurrants #
Rhubarb
Rice (must be brown)
Roe

S
Salad cream (very small amounts)
Salmon
Sardines-?
Scallops
Seakale
Shellfish
Shrimps
Skate
Sole
Spinach
Spirulina
Sprats
Squash

Squid
Steak-?
Strawberries #
Suet-?
Sultanas #
Sunflower seeds
Swedes
Sweet corn
Sweet potato
Sweets #

T
Tomatoes
(be wary of)
Tongue-?
Tripe-?
Trout
Tuna
(drain brine or sunflower oil)
Turbot
Turkey (no skin)
Turnip

V
Veal-?
Venison -?

W
Walnuts
Watercress
Whelks
Whitebait
Whiting

Y
Yam
Yoghurt
(PLAIN LIVE ONLY) one serving every day, very little if extreme intolerant. Or take pro biotics.

Anything without a symbol, you can eat in the most part as much of as you like, especially all the greens, white fish and brown rice, if rice affected you then it will not once recovery is under way.

Greens
Greens are very important especially broccoli, cauliflower, Brussels sprouts, cabbage, peas, carrots, runner beans, lentils, they help to heal the digestive tract, and a selection of vegetables must be eaten every day, this is vital for recovery, try steamed vegetables, the body breaks them down much more easily, and more of the nutrients are retained in them.

Bio Yoghurt
PLAIN LIVE, or PLAIN BIO yoghurt must be used because this has live bacteria in it, and is different from dairy products, in that its structure has been changed slightly, the lactose (milk sugar) has been converted to lactic acid by the bacteria, and thus it should not affect you if you have yeast overgrowth, although you should not have too much, no more than one serving every day.
This is very beneficial for recovery, and a good source of the B2, B6, calcium and vitamin A

In extreme intolerance cases even the live yoghurt may affect you, in which case you would be advised not to take the live yoghurt, and take pro biotics instead, as prescribed by your local health shop.

Do not take live yoghurt and pro biotics together, always take one or the other, or in some cases it could give you constipation.

Meats and Protein
The meats chicken and turkey, are lean meats, and very friendly and easy to break down vital protein, you can eat these as much as you like.

Lentils are a good source of vegetable protein.

You can eat steak but in small amounts, remember it's oily and fatty.

You can eat oily fish, but again in very small amounts, these are also oily and fatty.

Diet Relating To The Recovery Programme
I would advise everyone to start by not eating any of the foods listed on pages 42-45, or refer to the cut out wall chart on page 14, this includes the foods listed under, OTHER INTOLERANCE FOODS.

After the first two weeks, try introducing the foods listed under the heading OTHER INTOLERANCE FOODS, (refer to page 45, or the bottom of the cut out list on page 14) if you don't react to these foods you will be all right to eat them throughout recovery.

Eggs are one of the foods under the OTHER INTOLERANCE FOOD HEADING, people are usually ok with eggs once they have starting the diet, occasionally people react with them in the early stages of recovery, but this intolerance should diminish after two or three weeks on the diet.

Occasionally tomatoes react with people when starting the diet, it may take 6 to 8 months and several gallbladder and liver flushes before this intolerance subsides.

Virtually all food intolerants cannot cope with oranges, usually for about two years, and many gallbladder and liver flushes.

If you are extremely intolerant then you will have to start by eating only the greens, and apples pears and bananas, non-oily fish that carry no symbol, and chicken.

Also if you are extremely intolerant, you will have to completely stay away from anything with the -? next to it in early recovery, This is necessary to keep your digestive tract stable because extreme intolerants cannot break down oils and fats efficiently, until they have begun to flush the liver, after the first two or three flushes small amounts of the oily and fatty foods may be eaten, and then larger and larger amounts as you progress in recovery.

If yeast overgrowth is present which it usually is, then you will have to continue to stay away from all those items with a # symbol next to them, for at least 2 months and if you are extremely intolerant up to 12 months. It may be 18 months to two years, before you have beaten yeast overgrowth fully, and can have all of the fruits carrying this symbol # in large amounts. After about 2 months of recovery try eating peaches, apricots, etc if tinned make sure they are in their own juice and not in syrup, and monitor the effect it has on your digestive tract, if they bloat your stomach they will be feeding your yeast overgrowth, so eliminate them from your diet again.

SELF HELP

There is a great deal of self help required in some cases in very early recovery, you must listen to your body and take note of your reactions to ingested foods, it is unusual to find someone who is intolerant to any of the foods not carrying a symbol, but this does occasionally happen.

If the small quantities of oil give you stomach discomfort, then there is a very strong possibility you have gallstones, and you will have to complete a series of gallbladder and liver flushes.

Garlic and onions are detoxifiers and should be used in very small quantities in the early stages of recovery, and increased, as recovery progresses to help detoxification. Too much garlic or too many onions too early, will make you feel ill, because your detoxification system cannot cope with the toxins the garlic or onions have released, when it kills off the yeast overgrowth.

Sugary Products = Feeling Very Hungry.
In the first month or so of recovery you will feel very hungry, this is partly because your stomach will have to shrink down, after being swollen due to the inflammation caused by your food intolerance, and initially it will be like an empty cavern, you will not be breaking down and absorbing many elements correctly, and thus you will be short of many nutrients, this will make you feel hungry in the early stages of recovery.

Also if you eat any refined sugar or anything sweet, or drink alcohol it will make you feel very hungry, this is not a natural hunger but a desperate hunger, so keep away from these items, and you will only have what I call a natural hunger.

Other Reactions

If you still get a reaction after starting the diet, then you are either extremely food intolerant, or more it is more likely that you are inadvertently ingesting some wheat, so scrutinise everything you eat, and be certain that you have excluded all the possible sources of wheat, and any other possible reactive foods such as dairy products, Soya, orange, melons, stearic acid, lemons, sesame seed, and possibly eggs or even tomatoes.

Good advice when starting the diet is not to eat anything processed, do not eat packaged or tinned foods, i.e. free from biscuits and cakes, then you can be sure that you are not inadvertently eating anything you may react with.

With regard to the vegetables, these are much easier for the digestive tract to break down and absorb especially if they are steamed rather than boiled to death, it is extremely unlikely that you will react to any vegetables at all.

Obviously people vary slightly, so take note of your reactions to the foods you eat, on rare occasions people react to some of the foods in the list of foods you can eat, like nuts, this is very unusual and often the reaction goes away after some time into recovery, usually after any gallbladder and liver flushes required.

The primary and trigger intolerance, wheat, and the secondary intolerance dairy, are the main foods to stay away from.

If you have not become extremely food intolerant then you may find you can eat small quantities of oats, and some other of the reactive foods without reaction, but initially wheat and dairy products should always be avoided.

SO LISTEN TO YOUR BODY and the reactions you may have to ingested food.

Note

Occasionally some people have a slight intolerance to nuts and will have to avoid them until recovery is under way.

Some people have a definite allergy to nuts, or shellfish, which is a different kind of reaction, an allergic antibody reaction, and not intolerance, there is an important distinct difference between the two reactions, and they should not be confused with each other.

This kind of reaction is an allergic one, and can lead to your body going into anaphylactic shock.

People often confuse the two, so I thought I would make it clear that we are dealing with intolerance in this book, and not allergy.

Obviously if you have a nut allergy, you will know full well the consequences of ingesting these products.

POSSIBLE FOODS FOR EACH MEAL

So what could you put together as a meal, first I'll just give you a few possible foods for each meal? There are some recipes later in this chapter.

Foods For Breakfast:
• Apple

• Bacon
  (small amounts at first and grilled)

• Banana

• Coconut milk

• Egg boiled, scrambled, or poached
  (with rice milk, try them and gauge the reaction after 2 weeks on diet)

• Gluten free crispbread

• Gluten free porridge
  (available from supermarkets)

• Grapefruit
  (in own juice, small amounts)

• Herbal drink

• Home made potato cakes

• Mackerell
  (drain off brine or sunflower oil, in small amounts)

• Nuts or sunflower seeds

• Pear

• Pineapples
  (in own juice, small amounts)

• Prawns

• Rice brown

• Rice milk

• Scrambled eggs and salmon flakes

- Smoked haddock

- Tomato
  (beware tomatoes in early recovery)

- Tuna
  (drain oil or brine)

- Vegetables
  (any of them)

- Yoghurt
  (must be plain live - only at one meal every day)

Morning Or Afternoon Snack:
- Apple

- Banana

- Biscuits
  (coeliac, wheat, soya, dairy, sugar free)

- Carrot

- Celery

- Nuts or sunflower seeds
  (not in early recovery if you have diverticulitis)

- Pear

- Tomato
  (beware tomatoes in early recovery)

Foods for lunch:
- Apple

- Baked beans
  (in small quantities, they may contain sugar, and possibly gluten)

- Banana

- Beef
  (small quantities in early recovery)

- Coconut milk

- Chicken

- Chips
  (occasionally, if frozen check for wheat coating)

- Corn based pasta
  (corn and vegetable based available in most supermarkets)

- Lentils

- Mayonnaise
  (very small amounts in early recovery)

- Nuts or sunflower seeds
  (not in early recovery if you have diverticulitis)

- Pear

- Brown Rice

- Rice cakes

- Rice milk

- Salad dish
  (onions help detoxify, not too many in early recovery)

- Vegetables
  (any of them)

- Yoghurt
  (must be plain live, only at one meal every day)

Try mixing any of the following, your favourite vegetables, beans (not tinned in tomato sauce) rice, tuna, beetroot, prawns, onions, a dash of ginger or herbs, live or bio yoghurt, for a lunch box to take to work (very little or no mayonnaise in early recovery, it has vinegar in it, it's too oily and fatty and may contain wheat,) This or variations on this theme is what I usually take to work every day along with some fruit.

Ginger or peppermint is excellent for soothing the digestive tract.

Foods For Dinner:

- Apple

- Banana

- Chicken

- Chips
(occasionally, beware of in chip shops, they may be fried in wheat gluten contaminated oil, and frozen chips from supermarkets may contain wheat)

- Corn based pasta
(made from corn and vegetables available in most supermarkets)

- Egg dish

- Fish
(non oily fish in early recovery)

- Grapefruit
(in own juice, small amounts)

- Pear
(in own juice)

- Pineapple
(in own juice, small amounts)

- Potatoes
(mashed, boiled or jacket)

- Red meat
(small amounts in early recovery)

- Rice, brown. Plus Rice cakes

- Salad dish
(onions help detoxify, not to many in early recovery)

- Sausages - organic wheat and soya free variations

- Vegetable soup home made (watch the ingredients)

- Vegetables

- Yoghurt - plain live variants. Only at one meal per day.

SOME OF MY RECIPES

The following few pages are filled with some suggestions and recipes that may help to get you on the right track, although in early recovery (the first month or so) you will have to eat very basic food, salads, boiled potatoes, brown rice, lots of vegetables, and the allowed fruits.

In the first month or so of recovery don't eat anything processed, you need to know exactly what you are eating, the minute you open a tin or packet you have just lost control of your diet.

After the first month or so you may then try some recipes from gluten free books, and dairy free recipe books, but BE CAREFUL WITH THE INGREDIENTS, and make sure they don't contain any of the foods you cannot eat, for example, wheat, dairy, sugar, and possibly some of the OTHER INTOLERANCE FOODS orange, melons, lemons, Soya etc, these are listed on pages 43 to 46, or refer to the cut out wall-chart on page 14.

At least referring to some of these books will give you the choice of thousands of recipes, where I would be giving you maybe twenty.

You may be able to modify many slightly to fit your needs, this could be quite exciting if you consider yourself a bit of a chef, think of all those original recipes you could invent.

I would advise you not to use salt or pepper or any spices in very early recovery.

I know this may be a little boring, but initially very simple recipes are necessary to stabilise your digestive tract before you have claensed your liver.

After 2 or 3 flushes you will become less intolerant and will therefore be able to eat more and more of the oils and fats and forbidden fruits.

BREAKFAST RECIPES

Be wary of breakfast cereals, most are very high in sugar, and many contain gluten, such as corn flakes and rice based products.

RICE PORRIDGE

- Take some pre cooked brown rice from deep freeze and thaw out and heat.
- Take two dessert spoons of mixed herbs or spices (of your choice) and boil in 150ml of water, keep lid on pan to prevent water from evaporating.
- Take 100ml of coconut milk, if the coconut is in a set form take 1 heaped dessert spoon full and add 100ml of water
- Add 1 heaped dessert spoon of corn flour
- Strain water from boiled herbs into coconut and flour mix
- Heat mixture until it thickens
- Add in pre heated brown rice
- Add level teaspoon of honey
- Serve in bowl as porridge

GLUTEN FREE PORRIDGE

● Obtainable from supermarkets, make with rice milk, instead of cows milk.

MORNING SALMON

(Or any non oily fish)

● Chop lots of lettuce, watercress, celery, and grated carrot.
● Mix with fresh or tinned salmon.
● Moisten with live or Bio yoghurt.
● Sprinkle with very small amount of black pepper.

HADDOCK A.M

● Poached eggs and smoked haddock, (not too much haddock)

BANANA SMOOTHIE

(If you don't react to live yoghurt)

● 1 banana
● Tipped with live or Bio yoghurt (unusual for live yoghurt to react)

PRAWN A.M.

● One or two handfuls of prawns
● Chop some lettuce, watercress, radish, and celery.
● Mix with one tablespoon of Live or Bio yoghurt, (unusual for live yoghurt to react)

BACON AND EGG

(Try after first two weeks of recovery)

● Grill the bacon.
● Poach the eggs, or scramble the eggs in rice milk.
● You may try gluten free sausages, if you can source them, but only have one, they are potentially oily and fatty.

CHOPPED VEGETABLE OMELETTE

(Try after two weeks of recovery)

● Whisk two eggs.
● Heat small amount of oil in frying pan.
● Add eggs, spreading over base of pan, keep mixing all the time until cooked and transfer to plate.
● Add favourite pre cooked chopped mixed vegetables to top of eggs.

EGGS

(Poached or boiled, try after two weeks of recovery)

• May be eaten with gluten free crispbread

GRAPEFRUIT CRUNCH

(Unless extremely intolerant)

• Grapefruit, fresh or in own juice.
• Topped with live or Bio yoghurt.
• Sprinkle with chopped nuts, any of the following, brazil, almonds, cashew, walnuts, almonds, hazelnuts, or any of your favourite nuts, (no nuts if you have a nut allergy or diverticulitis)

PINEAPPLE CRUNCH

(Unless extremely intolerant)

• Pineapples, fresh or in own juice.
• Topped with live or Bio yoghurt.
• Sprinkle with chopped nuts, any of the following, brazil, almonds, cashew, walnuts, almonds, or hazelnuts, or any of your favourite nuts,
• No nuts if you have a nut allergy or diverticulitis

SARDINES AND TOMATOES

(Drain oil, but only if tomatoes don't react with you)

TUNA

(Drain oil or brine, with tomatoes, only if tomatoes do not react with you)

SALMON

• Cook a salmon, and spread the flakes on some scrambled eggs
• Add some chives to taste.

LUNCH RECIPES

JOHNS LUNCH

(May be eaten at any stage throughout recovery, may be eaten hot or cold)

Ingredients
• You may use pre packed frozen chopped vegetables.
• Your favourite pre cooked vegetables (pre cook freeze enough to last for a week at work)
• Plain Live or Bio Yoghurt (unless extremely intolerant)
• Tuna or any non-oily fish of your choice.
• Ginger
• Chop a stick of celery
• Brown rice, pre cooked (you may pre cook and freeze, make enough to last for a week at work)
• Beetroot

Method
• Take some of the pre-cooked vegetables.
• Add some of the pre-cooked brown rice.
• Add as much of the tuna or non-oily fish of your choice.
• Add the chopped celery.
• Season with pinch of ginger (salt and pepper later in recovery)
• Add live or B.I.O yoghurt.
• If you would prefer this to be hot then do not add the yoghurt until you have heated the vegetables rice and tuna, or the yoghurt will curdle.
• You may add onions after the first month of recovery.
• A little mayonnaise may be added when recovery is underway.

MIXED SALADS

(Can be eaten at any stage throughout recovery, you may introduce onions after first month of recovery)

You may make this a ham, beef, chicken, prawn, turkey, tuna, cottage cheese, or white fish salad, but in the case of the ham and beef only have small amounts of them until two or three gallbladder and liver flushes have been completed.

You may use
• Lettuce, any variety
• Celeriac
• Celery
• Watercress
• Radishes
• Beetroot (in own juice)
• Tomatoes (if you don't react with them)
• Melon (if you don't react with them)
• Cucumber (if you don't react with them)
• Sweetcorn tinned

Try adding the following sliced pre cooked vegetables
- Carrots
- Potatoes
- Sweet Potatoes
- Cabbage
- Parsnip
- Turnip
- Swede
- Peas
- Broadbeans
- Broccoli
- Cauliflower

You may use nuts
- Cashew Nuts
- Almonds
- Walnuts
- Brasil Nuts
- Peanuts (not salted)
- Hazelnuts
- Monkey Nuts
- Pistachio Nuts

Tips
You may add some apple sauce but remember with no added sugar.

You may add Live or BIO yoghurt (unusual for it to react)

You may add the following fruits
- Sliced apple
- Sliced pear
- Sliced banana.
- Avocado (in small amounts)

CABBAGE POTATO

(A very simple meal for the very intolerant)

- Steam or boil half a chopped cabbage
- Boil as many potatoes as you require
(Serve without salt or pepper in early recovery)

OMELETTE

Ingredients
- Ham
- Potatoes
- Mixed Vegetables
- Cottage Cheese

Method
- Break eggs into bowl and whisk.
- Select pre cooked vegetables, ham, grated cheese, or pre cooked potatoes.
- Cook in frying pan.

SOUPS

Ingredients
- Vegetable broth (home made),
- Chicken
- Lentils

Method
- When making home made soups use rice milk, and cornflour to thicken soups.

RICE CAKES OR GLUTEN FREE CRISPBREAD

Ingredients
- Spread with cream cheese
- Peanut butter
- Cottage cheese
- Tuna

DINNER RECIPES

JACKET POTATOES WITH VARIOUS FILLINGS

(Can be eaten throughout recovery)

Method
- Bake or microwave your potatoes until cooked
- Cut in half and scoop out potato and mix with tablespoon of rice milk, or 1 tablespoon of live or BIO yoghurt
- At this stage you may add your favourite filling to the potato, tuna, sweetcorn, mixed herbs, chicken, small amount of ham.
- After first couple of weeks of recovery try breaking an egg into the top of the potato and putting it back into the oven for 5 minutes to cook the egg.

CHICKEN RICE VEGGIE

For 4 people
(This meal may be eaten at all stages of recovery, yes I know it is a little bland but it will not upset your digestive tract, if you are extremely intolerant)

Method
- Place 3 to 4 lb chicken in oven 180 deg C / Gas Mk 4 for at least one hour until cooked through.
- Boil 6 oz of white rice for ten to fifteen minutes, until soft.
- Heat a selection of mixed pre chopped or frozen vegetables
- Mix some of the chopped chicken, white rice and vegetables.
- Serve as required.

BEAN SOUP

Serves 3
(After first month of recovery because of garlic and oil)

Ingredients
- 4 oz (110g) of dried white haricot beans, soaked in cold water overnight.
- 1 tbsp olive oil
- 1 garlic cloves chopped
- 1 ½ tablespoons chopped fresh parsley
- Extra olive oil to garnish (be sparing with oil)

Method
- Rinse the beans
- Put the beans in a large saucepan cover them with two pints of water and bring to
- Boil and simmer, half covered for two hours.
- Remove half the beans and blend in a food processor with a little of the liquid
- Return to pan
- Heat the olive oil in a small pan, add garlic and fry until soft
- Stir in parsley and then add to soup
- Pour into soup bowls and drizzle over a little olive oil and serve.

ROAST CHICKEN DINNER

(This meal may be eaten at all stages of recovery, N,B make sure that any gravy is thickened with cornflour)

Method
- Place 3 to 4 lb chicken in oven 150 deg C / Gas Mk 2 for at least an hour until cooked through.
- At last hour of cooking, place a tray using the fat from the chicken in the oven to heat up, when hot add potatoes and cook, turning regularly until browned and cooked through.
- Heat desired vegetables on top of stove, do not boil.
- Core and chop cooking apples, cook until mushy, do not add any sugar.
- Serve with gravy from chicken thickened with cornflour.

STEAMED FISH

(You may find this a little flat without butter, but you can eat as much of this as you like from day one of recovery)

Method
- Take any non-oily fish, filleted
- Take as many potatoes as you like
- Take as many mixed vegetables, as you like.
- Season with herbs (leave out salt and pepper in early recovery)
- Steam the fish until cooked through.
- Serve with boiled potatoes and desired mixed vegetables.
- Sprinkle with mixed herbs.

LANCASHIRE HOTPOT

Serves 4
(Because of onion content may only be eaten after first month of recovery)

Ingredients
- 1lb (450 g) middle neck of lamb
- 1oz (25 g) corn flour
- Small amount of salt and pepper
- 8oz (225 g) sliced carrots
- 4 Sliced onions
- 1 ½ lb (675g) sliced potatoes
- ¼ Pint gluten free beef stock

Method
- Heat oven to 450 deg F / 180 deg C / Gas Mk 4.
- Coat lamb cutlets in seasoned Corn flour.
- Place the lamb, onions, carrots and potatoes I layers in a large casserole, finishing with potatoes.
- Pour in the stock.
- Cover the casserole and put in the oven for two hours.
- Remove the lid and cook for a further 30 Min to brown the potatoes.

VEGETABLE RISOTTO

Serves 3
(After first month of recovery, and after three or four flushes you may mix 1 oz of butter ant 2 oz of parmesan cheese at the end of this recipe to enhance the flavour)

Ingredients
- 1 Aubergine
- 1 Courgettes
- 2 Tablespoons of olive oil
- 1 Sliced onions
- 2 Crushed cloves of garlic
- Small amount of salt and pepper
- 5 oz or 135 g of arborio rice
- ¼ pint gluten free vegetable stock
- ½ pint boiling water

Method
- Slice and cube whole aubergine and courgettes into small pieces
- Heat the oil in an oven proof heavy pan with a close fitting lid
- Fry the aubergines courgettes onions and garlic for 3 minutes, until soft
- Add salt and pepper to taste
- Add rice and stir to make rice absorb flavour.
- Take pan off heat and add stock, then boiling water, do not let it stick to bottom of pan.
- Put lid on and place in oven at 150 deg F / 180 deg C / Gas Mk 4 for 45 mins

TUNA AND SWEETCORN PASTA

Serves 2 / 3
(After first month of recovery or you may not be able to tolerate until you have completed at least two flushes, and then with caution, may be topped with cheese and baked in later recovery)

Ingredients
- 130g tin of tuna flakes in brine
- 400g tin of tomatoes
- 1oz mixed herbs
- 1 small tin of Sweetcorn
- 1 Pack of CORN based pasta
- 1 Large onion.
- Garlic to taste.
- Rice vinegar

Method
- Begin by cooking the pasta
- Fry onions in sunflower oil
- Mix together and add tomatoes, sweetcorn, a teaspoon of rice vinegar, teaspoon of honey and mixed herbs.
- Heat through Serve with either, potatoes, salad or vegetables.

BASIC TOMATO SAUCE

(For those without tomato intolerance and only after three or four flushes.)

This sauce can be the basis of lots of dishes, it can be poured over meat or vegetables, or try mixing various beans or pulses with it such as borlotti or cannelloni.

Ingredients
- 1 large clove of garlic
- 2 tablspoons olive oil
- ¼ - ½ teaspoon of chilli flakes(depending on taste)
- 3 x 400g tins Italian plum tomatoes (not chopped)
- 2-3 tablespoons extra virgin olive oil
- 2 teaspoons dried oregano
- 1 handful fresh basil, marjoram or both, roughly chopped.
- Salt and ground black pepper

Method
- Gently fry the garlic with the olive oil in a thick bottomed pan
- Add the chilli, oregano and tomatoes and mix gently, do not break up the tomatoes
- Bring to the boil and simmer for 1 hour
- Cook slowly or tomato pips will be released making the sauce bitter
- After this stir up and chop up the tomatoes
- Add the fresh herbs and season to taste
Add 2 to three tablespoons of extra virgin olive oil

REAL PEA AND HAM SOUP

(With care this may be eaten after the first month of recovery, you may or may not choose to use ham or bacon, it is not essential to make the soup, you could just make it a pea soup with chicken stock)

Ingredients
- 1-tablespoon olive oil
- 1- large onion or leek, or half of each
- small bunch of flat leaved parsley, keep some for serving
- small bunch of mint, keep some for serving
- the ham bone from the shank or bacon ribs (optional, whatever you prefer, these may even be left out altogether)
- 1.2l, or 2 pints gluten free chicken stock, or ham or bacon stock, you can to use either/or.
- 150g 5oz peas
- 150g 5oz green split peas
- salt and pepper (optional, be careful with)

Method
- This will taste better if made with a ham shank or bacon ribs.
- You should boil the ham shank for 2-3 hours, and if you use bacon ribs they will
- Take about 40-50 minutes of boiling, top up with water if required

- Remove the rind and fat and throw away
- Remove the meat from the bone and break it up or throw it in the liquidiser, depends how rustic do you want your soup
- Heat the oil in a thick bottom pan
- Add the onion or leak, or both
- Cook gently for about 8 min until soft
- Tie the parsley and mint together
- Add to the onions and or leek along with the split peas
- Stir to coat them with the onion mixture
- Stir for a minute and then add the chicken stock and ham bone or bacon bones if desired or required
- You may replace some of the chicken stock with the ham or bacon stock if required
- Bring to the boil and simmer for 20 min
- Stir in the peas and cook for a further 20 min until peas are tender
- Remove the ham or bacon bones
- Puree the soup with a blender
- Season as required
- Return to pan and add ham or bacon and reheat gently
- Serve garnished with chopped parsley and mint

BRAISED PUY, LENTILS WITH GARLIC AND ROSEMARY

Serves 4 (may be eaten after first month of recovery, with caution)

Ingredients
- 55g 2oz panletta or bacon
- 34g 12oz of puy lentils
- 1 tablespoon olive oil
- 3 heaped tablespoons chopped fresh rosemary
- 1 red onion, finely chopped
- 350ml 1 ½ pts chicken stock (gluten free)
- 2 cloves of garlic, finely chopped
- 2 tablespoons extra virgin olive oil
- salt and black pepper, season to taste

Method
- Thinly slice the panaletta or bacon
- Give lentils a rinse using sieve
- Heat 1 tablespoon of oil in a thick bottomed pan and add the panletta or bacon
- Fry until slightly coloured and then add the garlic, onions and rosemary
- Cook for a further 2 min, then add the lentils and fry for about 1 min
- Add the stock, put the lid on and bring to the boil
- Simmer on the hob or in the oven at 160deg c, 310f, gas mk2 for 1 hour stirring occasionally
- After 1 hour most of the stock will have been absorbed
- Add 2 tablespoons of extra virgin olive oil
- Season to taste

WHAT CAN YOU EAT AFTER FULL RECOVERY?

You may eat any of the foods listed or discussed in this chapter in any amount at all after full recovery, this also includes any of the foods in the "foods that can be eaten" list on pages 48 and 49, or the pullout wall chart on page 15.

Fruit and vegetables are an absolute must, and must be eaten every day.

Meat, even oily and fatty meats may be eaten, but if you are eating oily or fatty meats such as steak, try to eat them cooked rare or medium rare, you can eat a large amount at one sitting with no ill effect, this will also help to keep the liver clean, don't spread oil and fat throughout the day, there is nothing wrong with red meat, or oil and fat once you are fully recovered, your body requires oils and fats, and is naturally adapted to break down oil and fat and utilise them.

You may eat small amounts of dairy products, but not every day.
You may eat small amounts of wheat based products, but not every day, the problem is that wheat based products are usually in a processed form and you need to stay away from processed food which contains many unfriendly elements.

You may eat small amounts of sugar, but remember if you eat a lot of sugar you will turn on the hunger neurons which will tell you that you are hungry, so I would advise you to try and stay away from processed sugar, also remember that you will be giving your body the glucose instead of extracting it naturally from the foods you eat.

By far the greatest freedom I have found after full recovery is that you can go to a restaurant and order anything on the menu, and it will not affect you, all right I know there may be sugar, wheat, dairy products, E numbers, flavourings, preservers, etc in enormous amounts, but when you are fully recovered you can allow yourself the pleasure of a meal out now and then, so don't be afraid of letting your hair down, when you go out for a meal, indulge yourself, its fine as long as you don't do it every day.

You will find that after full recovery you will be satisfied even after a small meal, you may not feel full in your stomach but your hunger pangs will recede, and you will feel satisfied, in other words you will have satisfied your hunger.

WHAT CAN I DRINK?

Alcohol

Well, lets get the bad news out of the way first, you shouldn't drink alcohol, it is an extreme toxin for your system to eliminate.

If you have to drink don't drink beer, lager or wine (it has a potential yeast and gluten or wheat carry over and contains carbohydrate) you can drink most distilled drinks, e.g. Whisky, Vodka, Gin, or even Brandy but be careful, and check with the manufacturer if possible, to see if any of the fermenting grain extract has been added back into the drink for flavouring, after the distillation process, but I repeat you should drink as little alcohol as possible, if you are going to repair your liver, pancreas and digestive system.

Wine

Don't drink wine if you have yeast overgrowth, 99% of intolerants have yeast overgrowth, the yeast overgrowth loves wine in particular, and feeds off it.

This includes red and white wine.

Tea And Coffee

Don't drink tea or coffee. Tea is acidic, and coffee is an oxidiser (it tries to break down tissue), many intolerants react quite severely if they drink coffee, it often triggers their digestive tract within minutes and can give them loose bowels within an hour or so.

Orange Juice And Oranges

Don't drink orange juice, or eat oranges, the acids and sugars will affect your digestive system.

Fizzy Drinks

Don't drink any fizzy drinks or canned drinks, these have all sorts of additives, especially aspartame, aspartame is a commonly used sweetener, and many doctors and eminent scientists are finding this to be a very toxic substance, and the body finds aspartame very difficult to eradicate.

Many fizzy or canned drinks contain sugar, and this will give the yeast overgrowth fuel that it thrives on, they will also blow you up and make the malabsorption in your digestive tract worse.

Soya Milk

Don't drink Soya milk, it is high in protein, many intolerants have problems breaking down this high protein, it may affect your digestive system.

Daily Drinks

Oh, brilliant I hear you say, it's enough not being able to eat some of my favourite foods, now I can't even have my favourite tipple.

But do not despair, below are many drinks you can have, and may even begin to enjoy.

The good news is that there are many drinks you have probably never tried, and could even get hooked on, such as some of the ones listed below.

Try and rotate the juices daily, to make it more interesting, but remember if you are very intolerant you will not be able to drink orange juice.

If yeast overgrowth is present then remember anything sugary will encourage the overgrowth.

Water (At Least 1 Litres A Day)
Try to keep yourself well hydrated, drink at least 1 litres of fluid every day, preferably water, many naturopaths advocate drinking at minimum of 2 to 2 1/2 litres of water a day, but I think this is excessive, the diet you will be eating contains much more fluid than you were taking on board with your previous diet, mainly from the fruit and vegetables that you will be eating, so you won't need to drink water like a fish to maintain hydration.

Water is the best drink by far. This helps to dilute toxins and flush them out your system, and it will also help your kidneys to detoxify.

Although I have to say that drinking too much water can be detrimental, as many athletes find out to their cost when running marathons, this is because there electrolyte levels can be upset, due to not having enough elements such as salt in the water they are drinking en route.

So don't start drinking litres and litres of water every day.

You may have lost your sense of thirst if you are extremely intolerant, if this is the case then just drink one litre of water or so a day, if your sense of thirst has not been affected then drink when you are thirsty, as nature intended.

Herbal teas
Many types, try some until you find one you like

Coconut milk
Very good for killing yeast overgrowth in the lower digestive tract, contains caprilic acid, it may affect extreme intolerants before they have done one or two gallbladder and liver flushes.

Ginger
A little ginger powder and oregano in a cup with boiled water settles the stomach

Mango juice
Small amounts, potentially very sweet

Oregano
Use Oregano from supermarkets, put in a cup of hot water and allow to steep for a couple of minutes, very good for killing back yeast overgrowth.

Pineapple juice
Contains some digestive enzymes and can be beneficial if drunk in very small amounts, no more than a quarter of a cup, with a meal, once a day, but beware, even this small amount may affect you, if you have been extremely food intolerant, but you should be ok with it after you have completed one or two of the gallbladder and liver flushes.

Rice milk
May be drunk or used as you like, I have never come across a reaction to rice milk.

Apple juice
Very good if gallstones are present, it helps to loosen them, drink in very small quantities, no more than a quarter of a cup, once a day, unless running up to a gallbladder and liver flush)

Grapefruit juice
Contains digestive enzymes, again in very small amounts, no more than a quarter of a cup, once a day, again if you are an extreme intolerant you may even be affected by this small amount, until one or two gallbladder and liver flushes have been completed.

Lemon juice.
A little in the bottom of a cup, top it up with water and drink, don't drink this in early recovery, it may react with you, until some gallbladder and liver flushes have been completed.

Cranberry juice.
Importantly make sure it is not sweetened juice, the trouble is that unsweetened cranberry juice is very difficult to find.

Very good for killing bacterial and fungal infections in the urinary tract, such as thrush.

Again drink a small amount of unsweetened cranberry juice, no more than quarter of a cup a day, you may be affected by even this small amount, until some gallbladder and liver flushes have been completed.

You are usually better advised to eat cranberries themselves if you have thrush, there is obviously nothing sweet in cranberries that can counteract thier effect, and feed the thrush.

Don't have all the fruit juices on the same day, your only allowed one a day, if on any one day, you drank a quarter of a cup of all of them, you would certainly have a reaction, feeding your yeast overgrowth, causing bloating.

ALCOHOLIC DRINKS

As I said before if you want to drink alcohol, then you may drink the ones listed below.
- Whisky
- Gin
- Vodka
- Brandy

After all you cannot be expected to turn into a hermit, and not let your hair down now and then. You will find that even these alcohols will affect your bowel movements, and stool colours, for up to 10 days after you have drunk them, but they will not make you feel extremely hung over and ill the next day, as would be the case if you drank beer, lager, or wine.

Your system can cope with whisky, gin, vodka and brandy far better, they are much cleaner, with far less chemicals in them for your detoxification processes to deal with.

Remember, any beer, lager or wine will feed your yeast overgrowth.

So be very careful about what you drink,

Motto; "THINK BEFORE YOU DRINK"

SOUPS OR BROTHS AS A DRINK

You can make yourself some very good soups or broths, if you are prepared to spend a little time making them.

Below are a few suggestions for making broths, or you can conjure up your own recipe.
You can experiment with the following using different combinations of vegetables and seasonings until you arrive at one you like.

THE BASIC RECIPE FOR MAKING A BROTH

Ingredients
- ½ litre of water
- About 3 mugs full of chopped mixed vegetables as required
- May include: Carrots
- Potato (including, peelings)
- Beetroot,
- Celery,
- Peas,
- Cabbage,
- Beans,
- Cauliflower

- You may want to add in something to season it, such as:
- Fresh Thyme
- Onion,
- Garlic,
- Parsley,
- Ginger,
- Mint,
- Basil,
- Sage

Method
- Put your chosen ingredients into a blender for about 1 minute.
- Put in a saucepan and bring to the boil, and then simmer for five minutes.
- You can filter the fluid from the broth and drink it or drink the whole broth.

THE RECOVERY PROGRAMME

GETTING STARTED

First of all you will have to get your stall set out, go shopping and get all the products you are going to need to be able to comply with the diet. Refer to the list of foods you can eat on pages 48 and 49, or refer to the cut out chart on page 15.

Be careful when you buy your food, don't assume that the many wheat, gluten and dairy free foods will not react with you, some of these foods contain elements, such as sugar, preservatives or colourings, other than gluten or lactose, these added ingredients could cause a reaction and very often do. They may contain caffeine or raising agents, which may not be on the ingredients, but may also cause a reaction.

I would advise you only to purchase foods, which have not been processed, packaged, tinned or bastardised in any way, and then you can be quite certain that you are not inadvertently eating something that may cause a reaction.

If you try and start this programme without all the ingredients, you will inevitably fail to stick to the diet properly, in fact even if you have all the ingredients you will find it very difficult in the early stages, especially in the first month or two.

You need to take the advised supplements, such as zinc, folic acid, iron, pro biotics, vitamin E after a month into the recovery programme, try the supplements as detailed in the recovery programme instructions, one at a time to start with, and if any react with you try a different type, if any one of the supplements consistently affects you then stop taking it all together, the elements used to bind some tablets could be affecting you, be wary of stearic acid in tablets.

If you have stomach-ache and cramps all the time at two months, then it's a good idea at this point, to go to your doctor, and be tested for helicobacter pylori, and if it is present eradicate it, for further information refer to page 162.

Bear in mind that you will not fully recover, until you have completed all the gallbladder and liver flushes required to regain bowel function.

THE FIRST MONTH

We have to take the inflammation away first, and begin to get the yeast overgrowth to settle down on its own, so for the first two weeks or so you must try to get to grips with and adhere to the diet, not eating anything on the "foods that cannot be eaten" list on pages 42-45, or refer to the cut out list on page 14, after the first two weeks you can try the foods listed under OTHER INTOLERANCE FOODS on page 45, to see if any react with you.

Do not take any garlic, onions, or detoxifiers in the first month, this may kill the yeast overgrowth too quickly, creating toxins, overloading your ability to expel these toxins, and making you feel ill.

Stay off dairy products (except live yoghurt, but only one serving every day, if this small amount affects you then take a pro biotic preparation, instead of the live yoghurt, (dosage as prescribed by your health shop).

You should be able to resume taking the live yoghurt and stop taking the pro biotics after a few liver and gallbladder flushes. Do not have both pro biotics and live yoghurt together; Take either live yoghurt or pro biotics, if you have both together it may give you constipation, most people are all right with live yoghurt from starting the diet.

Initially you need to stay off all foods listed carrying the # symbol next to them, refer to "foods that can be eaten list on pages 48-49 or the cut out wall list on page 15.

You can eat very small amounts of the oily foods carrying the ? symbol next to them, on pages 48-49 or refer to the cut out wall chart on page 15.

Stay on the diet, with lots of neutral foods i.e. vegetables, and the allowed fruits, and non-oily fish, or chicken.

Don't be frightened of eating lots of the "foods that can be eaten", that have no symbol next to them, you can break them down, so eat as much of them as you like.

THE SECOND MONTH

If you still have stomach cramps or a gnawing feeling in your stomach it is advisable at this stage to go for a blood test for helicobacter pylori. Remember the WARNING, if it is found that you have helicobacter pylori and it is eradicated you will feel much better, do not assume you are cured, remember the Helocobacter Pilori had only multiplied as a consequence of your upset gut flora, its not the Helicobacter causing your problems.

It is now that you should do the BEETROOT kidney treatment for the first time, as detailed in the kidney cleanse on page 223.

I would advise you to read "the kidney cleanses" chapter starting on page 218, before doing the cleanse.

After this treatment.
● Start eating a little garlic and onions, or detoxifiers like Propolis or Oregano,

● Take some milk thistle (silybum marianum) every day for a month (available from health shops)

● Take an iron tablet EVERY OTHER DAY for four weeks, but never on the same day as the following vitamin E, if the iron reacts with you, then halve the amount you are taking. If you still react then stop taking the iron.

● Take, 400iu of vitamin E once every FOUR WEEKS, no more or it may give you loose bowels if you are extremely intolerant. This vitamin E, MUST NOT BE DERIVED FROM WHEAT, and not be taken on the same day as iron.

• Take folic acid B12 once a day.

• Take 15mg of zinc once a day immediately before food, this helps food absorption.

• Stay off all the foods listed with the hash # next to them on pages 48-49 or refer to the cut out wall charts on page 15.

• You may eat very small amounts of the foods carrying this symbol ? (potentially very oily) on pages 48-49, or refer to the cut out wall chart on page 15.

• Stay off dairy products (except live yoghurt, one serving every day, even extreme intolerants should be all right with live yoghurt at this stage, if you still cannot cope with the live yoghurt then take pro biotics instead, (as directed by your health shop) remember don't take both together.

• You should have worked out by now, if any of the OTHER INTOLERANCE FOODS react with you listed on page 45, or refer to the cut out wall chart on page 14.

• You can eat as much as you like of the foods that carry no symbol.

3 TO 12 MONTHS

• Most of the symptoms will have died down by 3 months.

• Take folic acid B 12 once a day.

• Take 15 MG of zinc once a day.

• Take 400iu of vitamin E once every FOUR WEEKS, or after each gallbladder flush.

• Continue with the garlic and onions and possible detoxifiers, Propolis or Oregano as before.

• You may eat very small amounts of the foods carrying this symbol, ? (potentially very oily) on page 48-49, or refer to the cut out wall chart on page 15.

• You may try a gallbladder and liver flush after the first two months, as long as the stomach bloating has settled down.

• Even if you don't have gallstone symptoms, you must do at least 3 gallbladder and liver flushes, if you begin passing gallstones then you must keep flushing, at about six weekly intervals, until you are clear of gallstones, this could take two years or even more.

• Refer to the gallbladder and liver flush chapter, starting on page 228, for detailed instructions on the flush.

• Try small amounts of the foods carrying this hash # listed on pages 48-49 and the cut out wall chart on page 15.

• Stay off any of the foods that reacted with you, under the OTHER INTOLERANCE FOODS heading on page 45, or refer to wallchart on page 14.

• Stay off dairy products (except live yoghurt, one serving every day) if you still react to the live yoghurt, which is very unlikely at this stage, then take pro biotics instead (as directed by your health shop) remember do not take both together, either take live yoghurt or pro biotics.

• You can eat as much as you like of the foods that carry no symbol.

12 TO 16 MONTHS

• Take folic acid B12 once a day.

• Take 15MG of zinc once a day.

• Take 400iu of vitamin E once every FOUR WEEKS, or after each gallbladder flush.

• Continue the garlic and onions and possibly detoxifiers, Propolis or Oregano as before.

• You will have done a number of gallbladder and liver flushes by now, and you should be beginning to absorb much better by now, and your stool colours should slightly be darker.

• You should be able to cope with more and more of the oily foods ? by now, don't eat too many at this stage.

• Eat small amounts of the foods relating to yeast overgrowth #.

• Stay off dairy products (except live yoghurt, one serving every day) you should not react to live yoghurt at this stage.

16 TO 24 MONTHS

• Take folic acid B12 once a day.

• Take 15MG of zinc once a day.

• You can STOP taking the vitamin E at this stage, unless you have done a gallbladder and liver flush, then take the normal 400iu after each flush.

• You may try dairy and wheat based products in small amounts now, but be careful with them.

• Continue with the live yoghurt.

• Continue with the garlic and onions, and possible detoxifiers, Oregano or Propolis as before.

• You may have been full of gallstones and may still be doing the odd flush at this stage, make sure you finish all the flushes required to clean the liver and gallbladder, this may take two years or even longer in advanced intolerance cases.

- Extreme intolerants can take 4 or even 5 years of flushes to clean their liver and gallbladder properly.

- You should be all right eating oily and fatty foods after all the gallbladder and liver flushes that you will have completed by now. Fish oil is especially beneficial because it contains omega 3 oils.

- It is now that you should repeat the beetroot cleanse for the second time on page 223, and after about another month, do the herbal kidney cleanse on page 224. You will probably be at about 20 to 24 months by this time.

- You should be all right with the foods relating to yeast overgrowth # by now, so try eating some and see, although you will probably have tried some by now anyway.

24 MONTHS ON

- In extreme cases, if you have had a very clogged liver, you may need to repeat gallbladder and liver flushes every two months or so, until you stop finding stones or chaff in your stools.

- I had a seriously clogged liver, I was the worst case scenario, and required many flushes over eight years at random intervals, if you are an extreme case, you may need many flushes over 4 or 5 years.

- You should have alleviated the yeast overgrowth problem now, and killed it off properly, so you will be able to eat all the fruits carrying the # symbol relating to yeast overgrowth, and should now be able to eat dairy products again, without any reaction, wheat products may still react slightly.

- You should now be able to eat oily and fatty products in normal amounts, with no reaction at all.

- You may take a multivitamin supplement now, but this should not be necessary because you will be breaking down and absorbing all the elements required in maintaining a healthy body, with the possible exception of some trace elements like selenium, and zinc, which are rare in our modern environment or to be more precise, soils.

- You may now stop taking any of the supplements listed in this recovery programme, and to a degree lead a normal life, small amounts of unprocessed wheat products can be eaten, but you should stay away from processed wheat products.

- Dairy products may now be eaten but don't eat too many.

- Remember too much wheat dairy and sugar based products are how you clogged your liver and became intolerant to foods in the first place.

- So that's about it, you should now have regained a new enthusiasm and vigour for life, good luck and good health.

ACKNOWLEDGMENT

Thinking back to my teenage years, I can remember that I always had problems with my tummy. Always feeling bloated after a meal and pain in my stomach as well has always having indigestion. Through the years I have tried all sorts of remedies for indigestion, but none really got to the bottom of the problem.

Now I am 48 years old, a woman, and about a year ago I started with severe pains in my stomach, always having heartburn and feeling nauseous. I really felt ill all the time. I went to the doctor and I had a blood test and they found I had Helicobacter, a bacteria that lives in the bottom of the stomach. The doctor gave me strong tables for a week, which I had to take strictly, and it cleared the condition. I kept on some milder form of tablets afterwards to help calm down the acid that I was making and also kept on a fat free diet. But I kept having stomach ache and indigestion together with a pain under my right hand side rib cage, so I went back to the doctor after feeling very nauseous. The doctor explained that the symptoms I was showing pointed to gall stones. I was sent for a scan, but no gall stones showed up. I thought I must be imagining the symptoms, so I ate normally, but I kept feeling bloated and heartburn was still a big problem and the pain was still there.

So I met John and all the symptoms that I had were just like John's, so I went on his wheat-free diet and after a week I felt not so bloated, only a slight niggling pain and definitely no heartburn, which was so different, it was heaven.

I felt quite light headed for about a week, but that cleared afterwards and I lost 1 stone in weight. I kept strictly to the diet because I wanted to get better, but still the niggling pain was there on my right side. After about two and half months on the diet John thought I was ready for the Liver Flush, so I followed the procedures of the flush and in the morning I was quite amazed at the numerous stones about the size of a fingernail and loads of white gravel and black grit that I passed.

THANK YOU, John.

L. M Jackson

Linda Jackson

WHAT HAPPENS IN RECOVERY?

Initial Advice

Before we start I will make it clear that you will not recover overnight, it may have taken thirty or forty years for your system to degrade to the point where you start thinking, this is not normal; so obviously you will not recover overnight, and a self determination has to be adopted if you are to conquer the food intolerance phenomena, and related problems.

You have to change your mindset, you are ill and the only way you are going to recover is to follow the recovery programme detailed in this book to the full, a half hearted attempt will make you feel better, but you will not recover fully, unless you follow the recovery plan to the full.

Where the diet is concerned, just keep saying to yourself, I am not on a diet, I am eating the foods my body has naturally evolved to eat, and can easily break down, it's the rest of the western world that's on a diet.

Once fully recovered you can eat all of the foods listed in the foods you can eat chapter, in any amount you like, even the ones carrying the -? and # next to them on pages 48-49 and the cut out wall chart on page 15.

The only true measure of recovery with this condition is; how do you feel. After all, when you went to the doctors and explained your symptoms, and possibly had numerous tests, you may have been told; "there is nothing wrong with you", or more to the point they could find nothing measurably wrong with you, they may even have said, "you may be depressed", or "it may be in your head", but, it is more likely that you will be diagnosed with IBS or ME.

For someone who has nothing wrong with them, you don't half feel ill when in the depth of food intolerance, and when starting this recovery programme.

Obviously we are all intolerant to differing degrees, and therefore you may not have all the symptoms as described in this book, subsequently I have to start with the assumption that you are very intolerant to cover the whole subject and every scenario, but you will be able to find yourself and your own level in this book somewhere.

You will very quickly learn that stepping off the recovery programme and eating some of the forbidden foods, especially wheat based products, or drinking the wrong drinks, will cause a reaction and make you feel very weary, bloated and uncomfortable, especially in early recovery.

FIRST TWO MONTHS

In the first two months the following symptoms will begin to ease.

• The aching joints and muscles will begin to ease.

• The loose bowels or constipation will begin to improve.
• Your gaseousness will diminish.

• Your bloated stomach will improve dramatically.

• The acid reflux will slowly disappear.

• Your sleep pattern will improve dramatically.

• Your flu like symptoms should ease.

• Your itchy rectum will go away.

• Your Anaemia will improve.

• Your energy levels will improve.

• Your headaches will ease or go altogether.

• Your bloated appearance (retention of fluids) will begin to diminish.

• Your yeast overgrowth will ease

• Your Spots or acne should ease.

• Your Light-headedness and tendency to faint easily should drift away.

• Your irritability will go away.

• The mucous in your eyes first thing in the morning will ease.

• Any roseacea (flushing red face) will go.

2 TO 12 MONTHS

Often there is so much bloating and inflammation of the digestive tract and organs, that other symptoms are being masked, and after 2 months or so of adhering to the advised recovery diet, you will either realise that other symptoms have been uncovered, such as the gallstone symptoms, or you will notice a marked improvement in your well being.

I have had many people who have been scanned for gallstones and told "you definitely do not have gallstones", but still have all the symptoms, so I persuade them to do a gallbladder and liver flush, and to their surprise they flush out hundreds of gallstones, and then the pain and symptoms begin to subside.

Remember a scan does not always find gallstones and definitely will not find a clogged liver, therefore at least 3 gallbladder and liver flushes are always recommended, and thereafter as many flushes as are required to clean the gallbladder and liver completely.

In many ways a scan is a little pointless, even if they find gallstones you are going to flush them out anyway with the flushes. Do not let them steal your gallbladder, unless it is infected or calcified.

It depends on how far down the intolerance chain you have gone. If you react to all the "foods that cannot be eaten" on pages 42-45 or the cut out wall chart on page 14, then you are extremely food intolerant, and are certain to have yeast overgrowth and a clogged liver, and you will have a much harder battle to regain full recovery, and a long and sustained battle will have to be waged to kill off the yeast overgrowth, as described in the yeast overgrowth chapter.

The best advice I can give you is to say to you, listen to your body and your reactions to ingested foods, and try to judge for yourself how you are recovering. I can only advise you, and wish I could be there to support you when you have off days, and when you cannot understand why you have had an off day, and feel worse.

For instance, if you try to kill off the yeast overgrowth too quickly with too much garlic, onions etc you will feel off, this is because you are killing off the yeast overgrowth, faster than your system can expel, and detoxify the toxins released by the dying overgrowth.

The following symptoms will begin to ease between two and twelve months.

• Any involuntary twitching of skin will go. (skin palpitations)

• The gritty eyes will improve.

• The intolerance of bright light will begin to ease.

• Any itching all over your body will go.

• You will find you have more energy as recovery continues.

• You will find you have far more breath when exercising.

- Your athlete's foot will ease

- Your anxiety should begin to diminish.

- Any anaemia will diminish.

- Any hypoglycaemia will improve with each flush.

- Any gout will recede

- Any piles will recede.

12 TO 24 MONTHS

Once any and all of the required gallbladder and liver flushes have been done, and the final kidney cleanses, then a slow and gradual improvement will be observed as the organs of the body begin to recover, and your digestive tract regains the ability to break down, absorb, and interact the many elements required to run your body at it's optimum.

After you have cleaned out your liver, and cleaned out your kidneys, you will notice a vast improvement in your stool formation, they will go darker in colour, and much more stable, this is a good sign that you are producing and freely passing more bile, hormones and enzymes, therefore your toilet visits will become much more regular, about once a day or even once every two days.

You may need to stay off the yeast overgrowth foods, for the remainder of your recovery or the last twelve months, to fully eradicate it and be certain you have conquered it, although once the gallbladder and liver flushes, and the kidney cleanses have been done the yeast overgrowth will die back dramatically, and usually stays away.

To be honest by this stage the best advice is to listen to your body, and feel your way tentatively, by introducing very small quantities of some of the foods you have been advised to avoid, and gauge your reaction.

Don't think I feel all fight now, after about 12 months, and begin to drift into eating large amounts of the foods you should not eat, or you will have a relapse and undo some of the good work you have done.

It will take some time before one or two of the other symptoms begin to diminish, possibly up to three years, especially if you have been extremely intolerant and it has taken two years of cleansing or even more, to recover your gallbladder and liver.

These late recovery symptoms include.

- Dry patches of skin will heal.

- Any aching gums and bleeding gums will go.

- Any oily skin will go.

- Any Impotency will begin to go away.

- Any sensitivity to fumes etc will go.

- Any excessive sweating will go.

- You will feel warmer on cold days, and keep cooler on hot days.

- Your nails will grow more rapidly.

- Improving energy levels.

- Lines on fingernails will diminish.

- Splitting fingernails will go.

- Thick toenails will go.

- Any fungal infections will die back and disappear.

- Your athletes foot will disappear completely.

The following is a list, and explanation of some of the reactions and noticeable improvements you may experience whilst advancing through recovery.

Headache
You may find that you have a headache for a few days when first starting the diet, this is quite normal and will usually pass after the first few days or at most a week or so.
Some people have intense headaches before starting the recovery programme, these will improve dramatically once on the recovery programme.

Acid Reflux
The acid reflux will go completely, or will diminish markedly after two to three weeks on the diet, and you will feel much more comfortable after eating, and far less bloated.

Hunger
One of the biggest problems in early recovery is hunger, but remember you can eat as much as you want of the foods that you can eat, so don't be frightened of eating.

The problem is you are not breaking down, or absorbing, all the vitamins minerals and nutrients required to run your body efficiently, so the neurons in your brain will continually keep firing and letting you know that you are hungry, hunger is a considerable problem in early recovery.

You will feel very hungry for the first month or so, there are two reasons for this, firstly your stomach will be like an empty cavern, after all that bloating in the depths of your food intolerance, therefore you will never fill it until it has shrunk down, which will take up to a year, plus if you are not absorbing and interacting foods properly in the early stages of recovery, this will leave you feeling hungry, because your brain will constantly be craving nutrients which it knows your body is lacking.

You will continue to be hungry until you have completed some gallbladder and liver flushes, and begun to absorb more of the nutrients your body requires.

Water
If you are extremely intolerant and bloated in appearance, you will pass and loose lots of water for the first few weeks of recovery, this is your body loosing its excess fluids, and water retention, due to an increase in osmotic pressures between body tissues.

Bloated Appearance
This is what I refer to as the Michelin man appearance. You will loose the bloating in your whole body noticeably over the first couple of months, and not only will you loose the bloating, but you will seem to shrink as well, this is due in some part to water retention, and the loss of fluids as mentioned before.

Weight
Your weight will fall quite rapidly at first as excess fluids and fat are lost, and then you will begin to stabilise at your optimum body weight.

The only exception to this is if you are an extreme food intolerant, then your weight may fall rapidly in early recovery, and then continue to drift down very slowly until well into recovery, then you will begin to put on weight again, and stabilise when you reach your optimum body weight.

If you are extremely intolerant the most noticeable and dramatic improvement will happen in the first two weeks, in my case I lost three inches off my waste, and lost about five pounds in weight!

Tiredness
The extreme tiredness will begin to go away more and more over the coming months of recovery, but in the first few months, you will have bad days and good days, on a bad day you may feel quite tired, and possibly exhausted, but on a good day you will have more energy and vitality.

This is because you may not be expelling toxins as fast as you are producing them, and not absorbing properly, but if you keep to the diet, keep treating the yeast overgrowth, do the gallbladder and liver flushes, and flush the kidneys, you will slowly improve, and have more good days than bad ones.

Exhaustion
In the early stages and in the depths of my condition, I found that I occasionally virtually collapsed, that is to say that I completely lost all my energy, even breathing became a task. Its like your whole body shuts down, this commonly is called ME or yuppie flue.

If you have never experienced this then you have no understanding of what I mean, if you have experienced this then you will know exactly what I mean, and understand the condition, this reaction should begin to fade away slowly, although you may still get the odd attack once every now and then, even for the first year or so, if you do get these attacks they will noticeably improve once you have completed the first two or three gallbladder and liver flushes.

This condition is definitely a reaction to your long-standing intolerance to food such as wheat and dairy products, which have clogged your system.

In the middle of recovery you will have off days, but as recovery continues there will be more good days than bad ones.

Aching Muscles, Back, Joints

Your aching muscles, joints and possibly lower backache will improve dramatically in the first few weeks of the recovery programme, because we have taken most of the toxic load off your system, and therefore you will be able to expel unwanted elements much more efficiently, which were interfering with the functioning of your muscles and joints.

Eyes

Your sensitivity to bright light will only improve after a few months on the recovery programme, and usually improves dramatically after a few gallbladder and liver flushes.

The gritty feeling in your eyes should improve after two or three weeks on the recovery programme.

Any stinging in your eyes will not fully go away until you have completed the recovery programme.

Gallstone Indicators

If you continue to have an upset and churning stomach after eating food, and continue to have loose bowels, within, and after the first eight weeks or so, it is a good indication that you have gallstones and your liver is very clogged, an early gallbladder and liver flush will be required, but try to leave the flush until you have stabilized your weight and lost your bloating and bowel inflammation.

This often takes about eight to twelve weeks, I have to say that this will be eight to twelve weeks of frustration, some people want to do a flush in the first week, but this is not a good idea, you need to control and stabilise your digestive tract first, and ensure that any inflammation within your digestive tract has subsided.

After being on the diet for two to six weeks, gallbladder symptoms may begin to appear, such as a dull ache under your right shoulder blade, aching in your right shoulder, or a dull ache just under your right ribcage, these symptoms were being masked by the inflammation and bloating, before you began the recovery diet.

Helicobacter Pilori

If after a month or so on the diet you still have stomach pains, and severe cramping as apposed to the aforementioned stomach churning and loose bowels, then I would advise you to go to your doctor and ask for a blood test for helicobacter pylori.

There is a reasonable chance you have the bacterium with this type of symptom, and it will have to be eradicated before we can resume recovery, the use of antibiotics at this stage is a disappointing setback, but you will have to do this before we can resume the recovery programme.

Again I will repeat a WARNING stated before in this book, if you have helicobacter pylori, and it is eradicated you will feel much better, do not assume you are cured, the only reason this bacteria took off in the first place, is because you have gained food intolerance and your liver is clogged, and your upset gut flora has allowed the Helicobacter to proliferate, therefore you must continue to follow this recovery programme.

Further information can be found in the helicobacter pylori chapter on page 162.

Anxiety And Memory

You may have had quite bad anxiety, worry, and cycling thoughts, with an inability to resolve problems in your mind, whilst in the depths of your food intolerance, but this will begin to diminish once you begin to recover, although it will not go completely until you are fully recovered.

If your name memory was affected it will improve dramatically as you advance in recovery.

Celiac

If you are a diagnosed celiac when starting the recovery programme, you will have been off wheat for months or possibly years, so you will be able to embark on the gallbladder and liver flushes much sooner than anyone starting from scratch.

If you have not been diagnosed as celiac, but think you may have developed the condition (diarrhoea and loosing weight) you should ask your doctor for a blood antibody, and biopsy of your jejunum to see if you have flattened villi, to confirm this, and make absolutely sure it is nothing more serious than celiac disease.

The antibodies in true Celiacs retain a memory against the gluten fraction of the wheat, therefore wheat and oats can never be eaten again without reaction, although I have to say that most Celiacs are not Celiacs, and have only gained food intolerance and flattened villi due to a clogged liver, and an inability to break down the foods they are eating.

Many celiacs can eat oats, with no reaction, if you are one of these people then there is a strong possibility that you are not actually a true celiac, and have been miss diagnosed, in most cases people who can eat oats and not wheat fully recover their villi after cleansing their liver and gallbladder, (technically if you are a true celiac you cannot eat gluten in bread and you would also react to the gluten in oats as well, and will never be able to eat these foods again)

Most of the population that have gained food intolerance, can be just as reactive to wheat and oats, with bloating and loose bowels, constipation, retention etc, but do not present with flattened villi or antibody reaction, these people are left in the IBS pigeonhole with no measurable symptom to define their condition, and are consequently left in medical no mans land.

Tingling Numbness And Dead Limbs

After a month or so the tingling and possible numbness in your fingers and usually toes will go or certainly diminish, and the dead limbs when sleeping should begin to ease and slowly drift away.

Urine Colour
A good indication of whether you are detoxifying and expelling toxins properly, is when you urinate, your waters should be slightly yellow. This is a good indication that your kidneys are detoxifying properly.

If your urine is very clear all the time, especially first thing in the morning, then you are probably not expelling toxins efficiently through your kidneys, other good indications of poor detoxification are aching joints, headaches, and aching muscles,

Kidney Flush
The first thing you should have done after adopting the diet is the first beetroot kidney cleanse, to clean out your kidneys, which will help in detoxification.

Gallbladder And Liver Flush
There will be a gradual and slow improvement in your condition, especially after you have done some of the gallbladder and liver flushes, marked improvements will be noticed if you found you had gallstones.

You may require a series of gallbladder and liver flushes, after each flush you would notice an improvement in your condition and well being, oily foods can then be eaten in larger and larger quantities over the next few months, as the liver recovers and rebuilds itself.

You will probably find that you will go from the original loose bowels or constipation, into a much more settled pattern, and visits to the toilet will become less frequent, and your stools will go firmer, you may even become slightly constipated for a month or so, after even one flush, usually at about two to three months into recovery.

Aches and pains in your stomach area will begin to fade away.

Any oily skin will improve once the gallbladder and liver is clean.

Yeast Overgrowth
You will find that the yeast overgrowth will die back markedly within the first twelve months. When yeast overgrowth is in its latter stages of dying off, you often find that you get a sore and dry throat for about two weeks.

This is the yeast overgrowth having one last attempt at taking over your system, and affecting your ability to detoxify, it could also be your thyroid gland or immunity in your throat recovering normality.

Once this passes then a noticeable improvement in your well-being will be observed.

Athletes Foot, Toenails
Any athlete's foot symptoms will begin to die back after you have completed some of the gallbladder and liver flushes.

It will take much longer for any thick toenails to begin to grow properly, this won't happen until you have completed the recovery programme, and then it will take a further six months for you to begin to absorb properly again, and rebuild your system, enabling your thick toenails to recover.

Temper

Many people say they become slightly aggressive and short fused in the first two weeks or so on the diet, you may also find that you are slightly aggressive, and short fused for a couple of days, after completing a gallbladder and liver flush.

Chinese medicine states that anger is stored in the liver, and therefore after a gallbladder and liver flush stored up anger may be released from the liver, and manifests itself in your mood, and actions over a few days after the flush, in some people there can be quite an intense reaction, I even had one client who would not drive for a day or so after a flush, because it made him feel so aggressive.

It is also partly due to an imbalance in the nutrients you are absorbing, at these differing stages in recovery.

The more you recover and the more you will become calm and controlled, and more placid.

I had the same response after the first two or three gallbladder and liver flushes, I once broke a light switch after it did not flick to the on position straight away, and I had to flick it again, I hit it out of frustration, this is out of character for me, as I am normally very placid, thank god the aggression only lasts for a day or so after a flush.

Feeling Cold

You may find as I did that you go through a period of feeling cold, as described in the cold phenomena chapter on page 192, this is usually after the first two months of recovery, and may last for a few months, if it is winter you will feel very cold, even if well wrapped up.

You will begin to feel warmer once your digestive tract begins to recover, and extract nutrients, your body will then be able to utilise this fuel, creating heat and keeping you warm.

Lines On Fingernails

It is only after the last flush required, that your fingernails will begin to grow more rapidly and the lines, and/or splitting running the length of them will grow out, and your nails will begin to shine and become more smooth.

Dry Patches Of Skin, Lips, Skin Palpitations, Itching

Stubborn dry patches of skin will begin to disappear, but only after you begin to absorb much better, this usually takes a few months and some gallbladder and liver flushes.

You will find that your dry bottom lip will only begin to go, once you have completed some gallbladder and liver flushes, your lips will then begin to go as soft as a babies bottom, and smooth and oily, and any dry patches at the corners of your mouth will also disappear.

Any intense itching will begin to diminish after about two months of recovery.

Any palpitations in your skin will begin to diminish after a few weeks on the diet, and will continue to go until you don't get any at all at full recovery.

Impotency

If you were extremely intolerant and had become impotent then you will begin to regain your abilities, you will regain the ability to raise and maintain an erection, and your sex drive will begin to recover, but this will only occur after the latter gallbladder and liver flushes.

Stool Colours

Stool colour is an extremely accurate and important indicator, it proves that you are regaining a free flow of bile throughout the entire liver and common bile duct, your stool colours will not be the very light colour they were in the depths of your intolerance, the bile enzymes and hormones will be interacting with the food you have ingested, at the correct time, peristalsis stabilises, activation of precursors improves absorption improves, thus stool colours change.

Below is a rough guide to indicate the colour your stools should be, if you are production and maintaining a free flow of bile enzymes and hormones down and through the common bile duct.

The colours below relate to different stages of recovery.

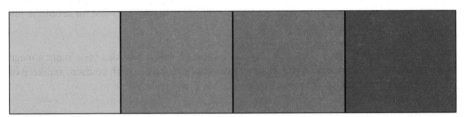

Too light   **Normal**

On the left is the light colour your stools will be in early recovery, and on the right is the colour they should be after recovery.

This chart is also on the rear cover of the book.

As I said before your stool colours will not improve too much until many or all the gallbladder and liver flushes required have been completed.

You will probably have completed all the gallbladder and liver flushes required after about 18 months to 2 years.

You will find that for a few days after a flush your stool colours may stay relatively light, until your gut flora recovers somewhat, then they will begin to darken, but as more gallstones begin to move out of the liver, and block your system again your stool colours will go lighter.

Sometimes, in the latter flushes your stool colours may stay quite dark, but if you flushed gallstones out on the previous flush, then you must keep cleansing until you stop passing gallstones.

You will learn to realise when you are beginning to block again, you will be able to feel a slight welled up feeling under your right hand ribcage, or a slightly full feeling in your stomach.

You may find that you block up again very quickly, especially when you get to the chaff stage in the latter flushes, in which case you will experience some discomfort around your midriff, and your stool colours may stay light after the previous flush, if this scenario occurs you will have to embark on another flush very quickly, often within 4 to 6 days, this is referred to as an emergency flush.

Finally

If you clean your system out properly with the gallbladder and liver flush, and the kidney cleanses, and eradicate the yeast overgrowth or Candida, do a bit of exercise, and eat the recommended diet, then there is no real reason why you should not make a full recovery, as long as permanent and lasting damage has not been done to your digestive tract.

It takes time to recover; after all you may be 50 or so as I am, remember it could have taken as long as 50 years of eating the wrong diet for you to descend into food intolerance, so patently you are not going to recover overnight.

The problem is often differentiating between some of the original symptoms, and the natural recovery symptoms, although the headaches, and stiff joints usually only last for about the first two weeks after starting the diet.

All your system has to recover and it takes time, there is no magic cure, this book is not a magic wand giving you instant recovery, therefore you have to be very strict with yourself, and keep on the programme until full recovery.

CAN YOU EAT WHEAT DAIRY AND OTHER PRODUCTS AGAIN?

The answer is almost certainly yes to dairy products, and yes to wheat products, if you clean your liver and kidneys and give them long enough time to recover i.e. two to three years.

The liver, gallbladder, pancreas, digestive tract thyroid etc, will repair and fortify themselves and you will begin to regain the ability to break down and process foods again, including wheat and dairy products, especially if your liver has been cleaned out properly as detailed in the gallbladder and liver flush chapter.

The intestine will regain the ability to break down, extract and to filter into your system the nutrients your body requires, and more importantly it will allow you to absorb the wide range of elements required in the correct balance, to run your body at its optimum.

After recovery you should try to eat a good diet, try to stay away from processed refined foods and refined sugar, try not to eat too many wheat or dairy products, then your body and more to the point your digestive tract will be able to maintain a healthy state, if you revert back to the diet you were on before starting this recovery programme, you will in twenty years or so be back in the same position, with gallstones and a clogged liver and impaired kidney, pancreatic and other organ impairment.

Another reason for staying close to the diet is the fact that you will be eating what you should be eating, in other words what your body has adapted and evolved to eat.

If you stay close to the advised diet you will also find it much easier to regulate your weight, and once fully recovered you will breakdown and absorb much better and put on weight more readily, but importantly if you stay on the diet you will find that you will easily satisfy your hunger without eating and eating, you won't feel constantly hungry.

Wheat Products
I suspect that very few people can be classified as wholly Celiac (someone who has flattened villi and igg or ige antibody reaction to gluten in bread).

Even some of the people who have these measurable scenarios, and gain intolerance to wheat in later life can still eat oats. This is odd because oats have a very similar gluten protein to wheat, and contain phytic acid, just as wheat does.Many celiacs are only celiac because their liver is clogged and requires cleansing.

So it seems that even those of us who are definitely not celiac, can be just as, or even more reactive to wheat than an actual celiac.

There is an excellent possibility that those of us without the measurable celiac condition, and just food intolerance, will recover to the point where we can ingest small amounts of unprocessed wheat products again, without any reaction.

The big problem with wheat products is the fact that you can only eat unprocessed wheat products, therefore you will find it virtually impossible to find something with wheat in it that has not been highly processed, when I say highly processed I mean made with high protein content flour, the flour they use for making bread, as discussed in the "what's wrong with wheat products" chapter on page 137.

I'm not saying you can go back to eating wheat products as you did before, if you did you may regain intolerance to it, but this would take a lengthy period of time, you will always be susceptible to eating large quantities of gluten over a lengthy period of time, especially if its in the form of modern fortified bread, it will slowly begin to clog your liver again.

Just for interest I walked down 5 isles of our local supermarket, and found very few products that did not contain wheat or flour of some sort, and these are products we purchase every day.

I cannot stress the wheat aspect enough, but by the time you get to this stage in this book you will fully understand how HIGHLY PROCESSED WHEAT reacts with you, after eating some, when I told you not to do in the early stages of recovery.

Wheat and what man is doing to it appears to be the trigger to all this, and when ingested in large quantities our systems cannot cope with it, especially after a lifetime of exposure.

Your body in the past was being saturated every day with this product, and could not cope with this barrage of wheat, gluten, etc every day.

Dairy Products

You will be able to eat dairy products again but only in small amounts and not every day. You should try to eat dairy products at just one meal, and not have small amounts at intervals throughout the day.

People like us patently have not developed the ability to break down large quantities of these products spread throughout our daily diet, and keep doing it over a number of years, without developing problems.

The problem has been to get your digestive system back into the condition where it can cope with these products again albeit in small amounts.

Dairy products will be all right in small amounts after about 14 to 16 months, however these may make you feel slightly tired after ingestion at first, because they are hard to break down.

Especially now that milk is pasteurised and the good bacteria has been killed off, along with the bad bacteria.

You will not have intolerance to dairy products once you have fully recovered. This intolerance was there as a consequence of the wheat intolerance, and a clogged up liver, and the consequential digestive imbalance.

Don't eat too many dairy products; they are too intense for people like us who are susceptible to over indulgence in these products.

Again if you go back to eating large quantities of dairy products they will imbalance your gut flora, and begin to clog your liver again over ten or twenty years, then you will have recurring symptoms.

Oats

There is a very good possibility that oats may be tolerated again with no ill effect, although they have a very similar gluten protein to wheat, and phytic acid in them.

They do not have the same reaction as wheat products; this is due to the fact that oats are far less intense than wheat flour, and are not fortified.

Some people find they don't react to oats even in the depths of intolerance, just as some celiacs can eat oats with no reaction.

You will have to try oats and gauge the reaction for yourself.

If you do react to oats you will tend to get a bloated stomach and it will make you feel slightly tired, although it may take 4 to 8 weeks for these symptoms to occur.

If you do react with them, remove them from your diet again and you will recover again over a few days or so.

Although I have to say that you are extremely unlikely to react to oats after full recovery.

Other Products And Receding Food Intolerance

Of the foods that are under the, other intolerance foods heading, in the foods that cannot be eaten chapter, on page 45 and the cut out wall chart on page 14, you will find that the egg, orange, lemons, Limes (citrus), sesame seeds, tomatoes, cucumber, and melon intolerances go first.

Then the Soya and then the dairy products, will go next, and all you're left with is the wheat intolerance, which should go completely once the liver is fully flushed and has had time to recover.

Don't eat too many Soya products, again small amounts is the thing.

You can drink orange juice again but don't start drinking gallons of it, small amounts and not often, if you want vitamin C eat some fruit and vegetables especially broccoli.

You will be able to eat melons, lemons, limes, sesame, and concentrated Stearic acid again without ill effect.

You will probably find you don't want to eat foods like wheat and dairy products much anyway, because you feel so much better on the diet you are on.

Obviously people vary and some people have not gone too far down the intolerance chain, and don't react to orange melons or Soya, and can always eat these with no reaction.

Remember if you eat anything with sugar in it you will feel hungry so stay away from sugar (processed sugar), the raw sugar will imbalance your gut flora, and microbial activity will be compromised, encouraging yeasts to flourish, this will diminish your ability to break down food.

You will also be putting your pancreas under stress, sending it on a roller coaster ride of insulin production.
Even the small amount of bread you may eat after full recovery will have sugar in it, so as I have said before I would advise you not to eat the processed bread again at all.

You would be better making your own bread from low gluten flour, and using sourdough, this bread will be harder than supermarket bread, but it will be much more friendly and easier to break down.

You will be able to eat oils and fats again with no reaction at all, there is nothing wrong with eating meats, your body has adapted and evolved over hundreds of thousands or even millions of years to eat meat, don't let anyone tell you that eating meat is not natural for human beings.

WHAT HAPPENS TO THE DIGESTIVE TRACT?

THE FAMILY TREE OF INTOLERANCE

Eating too much wheat gluten, dairy products and refined sugar.

Leads to imbalanced and distorted H.D.L, L.D.L and V.L.D.L

Leads to over production of cholesterol by the liver

- Cholesterol begins to coagulate in liver
- Impaired free flow of bile from liver.
- Developing gallstones.

Lack of bile Enzyme Production

- Upset gut flora
- Yeast Overgrowth
- Candida
- Helicobacter Pyori
- Bowel PH upset
- Peristalisis upset
- Digestive tract becomeds more porous

Become intolerant to food, mainly wheat and dairy products Lack of breakdown and absorption of foods, leads to.

- I.B.S
- Gallstones
- Thyroid problems

- M.E Yuppie Flu
- Chronic Fatigue
- Kidney Problems

If you still have a relatively free flow of bile from the liver

↓

Excessive Cholesterol enters digestive tract

↓

- Cholesterol is re absorbed adding to cholesterol already in blood. Leads to high cholesterol in blood.
- Clogging of arteries
- Heart Disease
- Heart Related Conditions

Celiac Disease
The Emergency State
Pancreatic Problems

- Stomach and Intestine Disorders
- Stomach Ulcers
- Ulcerative Colitis
- Chron's Disease

This is an extremely complex subject; some of this chapter will contain a theory of what I now believe to be happening to the digestive tract in the case of wheat and dairy intolerance.

The problem is that the human body is extremely complex, and millions of interactions are happening every second, and therefore unravelling the causal factors of food intolerance from a biological, or chemical perspective could be virtually impossible, because the balance of one element is obviously effected by other elements, therefore to try and correct the balance with say just one drug, vitamin, or mineral, may alleviate symptoms but does not address the cause or causes.

This is why it is often said that the doctor prescribed one or other drug, and took away the original symptom and gave me two others.

First we will have a brief look at how the digestive system works. In this chapter I will keep the explanations in laymen's terms.

A more detailed and in depth explanation of how the digestive tract functions, and the problems which develop within it, can be found in the chapter entitled "The in depth Medical explanations", starting on page 248.

THE MOUTH

If we refer to the to the diagram on page 105, food is taken in and chewed in the mouth, this is a very important start to the digestive process, the chewing of food and mixing it with saliva in the mouth is the most important first step in breaking down foods.

Saliva contains many elements, therefore chewing food properly before swallowing is extremely important.

THE STOMACH

The food is then taken down into the stomach, where it is further broken down by juices, and acids secreted from cells in the stomach wall, food can stay in the stomach for between two and six or even eight hours, the length of time it is held in the stomach is directly related to how difficult the food is to break down, and the efficiency of your digestive tract.

THE SMALL INTESTINE

Duodenum

Food then passes into the first part of the small intestine, the duodenum, which is about 40 cm long. This is an extremely important element in the digestive system. This is where bile from the liver and enzymes from the pancreas flow in, to aid digestion.

You have one opportunity to pass bile from the liver, and pancreatic juices from your pancreas, into your food, and it is at this point in your small intestine, any impairment in this free flow of bile directly impacts on your ability to break down the food you have eaten.

Many elements are absorbed here including fat-soluble vitamins A, D, E and K, the B vitamins, B1 Thiamine, B2 Riboflavin, and B6 Pyridoxine, Other elements absorbed are calcium, magnesium, iron, manganese, copper, zinc, vitamin C and fructose and glucose.

Jejunum

The next part of the small intestine is the jejunum, this is about 3 metres long and is where nutrients are absorbed, as in the duodenum the jejunum also absorbs the B vitamins, B1 Thiamine, B2 Riboflavin. Other elements absorbed here are folic acid, which is water-soluble, and the sugars, sucrose, maltose and lactose, and most proteins, which are broken down into amino acids, are also absorbed.

The jejunum is where a biopsy is taken to determine if the villi are lead flat, like a flattend corn field: if they are then you would be deemed to have celiac disease.

Ileum

The last part of the small intestine is the ileum, which is about 3.5 metres long, this is where vitamin B 12 Cyonocabalonin, cholesterol and bile salts are dealt with, amongst other elements.

THE LARGE INTESTINE

Ascending, Transverse, Descending And Sigmoid.

What is left then passes into the large intestine, the ascending colon, the transverse colon, and then the descending and sigmoid colon.

The large intestine is where everything that is left has to be dealt with before it is defecated. Up to one litre of water can be recycled every day in the colon. Foreign elements are also dealt with here.

Although some food and vitamins are absorbed in this area, mostly it is concerned with re absorbing water and eliminating things like dead cells and cholesterol. It's the last chance your body has of separating the good material from the bad, and when it is working efficiently it is very efficient in its purpose and leaves little waste.

RECTUM

What is left then passes into the rectum ready for elimination and defecation.

PERTALSISIS

Food is passed through the full length of the digestive tract by waves of muscle contractions, called peristalsis, the best way to explain this action, is to watch a snake when it swallows food, you can see peristalsis in action, the food seems to glide down the snake, these are actually muscle waves, one after the other, pushing the food along the snake.

This wave action can be upset by many things, and in this case by an intolerance to food. These waves should be regular and in sequence, to keep food flowing through the digestive tract smoothly, in those of us who are food intolerant this wave action can speed up or slow down, or even become random and sporadic, causing one contraction to run into another, like the concertina effect in a traffic jam on the motorway.

This concertina effect causes the digestive tract to become unstable, and adds to the already protracted state of events ensuing, this is due to the ingestion of the intolerance foods. Again it's the intolerance foods that are the causal factor in upsetting the peristalsis, and not upset peristalsis causing the problem.

THE DIGESTIVE SYSTEM (Figure 1)

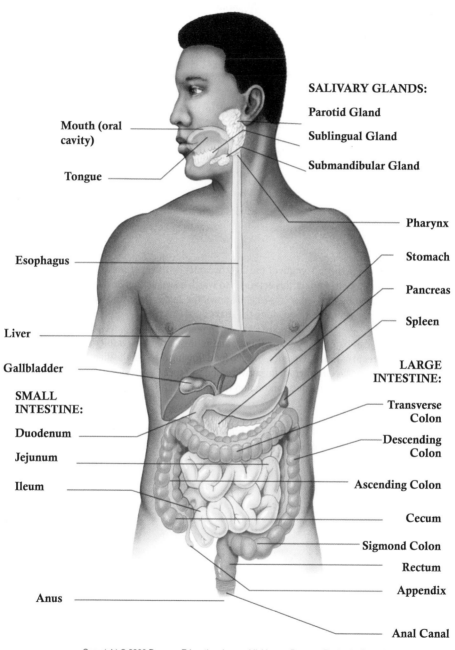

SALIVARY GLANDS:

Parotid Gland

Mouth (oral cavity)

Sublingual Gland

Submandibular Gland

Tongue

Pharynx

Esophagus

Stomach

Pancreas

Spleen

Liver

Gallbladder

LARGE INTESTINE:

SMALL INTESTINE:

Transverse Colon

Duodenum

Descending Colon

Jejunum

Ileum

Ascending Colon

Cecum

Sigmond Colon

Rectum

Appendix

Anus

Anal Canal

DEVELOPING PROBLEMS

There appears to be a very slow degradation of the digestive tract over a number of years with wheat and dairy intolerance.

In your younger years and through your youth you may not even realise you have a food intolerance at all, you may only have had vague symptoms such as constipation as a child, but your digestive system will have slowly been degrading, and trying to cope with what is obviously to us, too difficult a food to break down.

Our digestive tracts patently have not developed the ability over the few thousand years we have been ingesting wheat, sugar, and dairy products, to cope with the intense barrage, and more to the point over the last 50 years, a fortified intense barrage of wheat, sugar, and dairy products every day.

Our food is breaking down our digestive tract, instead of our digestive tract breaking down our food.

ACID REFLUX

Acid reflux is a consequence of ingesting too many processed products over a lifetime.

Your digestive tract responds very quickly after ingesting food, within twenty minutes it knows if it can cope with the food you have eaten, and will begin to respond accordingly depending on the type of food you have eaten.

If your digestive tract cannot break down the foods you are eating due to a lack of bile, enzyme and hormone production, then nature takes over and compensates by producing copious amounts of stomach acid, to try and help break down the more intense foods you have eaten before they move down into your intestine.

Excess acid production causes acid reflux and bloating, your stomach lining literally becomes slightly inflamed.

This reaction will diminish very quickly once the hard to break down intolerance foods are removed from your diet, the foods you will be eating on the advised diet are easily broken down by your digestive tract, thus your stomach will not be triggered into producing lots of acid, therefore the bloating and acid reflux will be controlled, without redress to medication such as antacids or acid blockers, or protein pump inhibitors.

Once we have recovered slightly, and bile and enzyme production has improved we can then tolerate small amounts of wheat and dairy products without producing excess stomach acid, unless you are extremely intolerant in which case even a thimble full of wheat or dairy products will affect you.

In the vast majority of cases (98%) a series of liver and gallbladder flushes are required, before you can eat wheat and dairy products again with no reaction at all, and to carry you through to full recovery.

BOWEL REACTIONS

In those of us who are susceptible the digestive system appears to run relatively normally for the first 15yrs or so with relatively normal bowel movements, then it begins to very slowly loose the ability to break down foods properly.

Often you don't notice too much in your middle years, but after a prolonged period, usually in your late thirties or early forties you may begin to experience a period of normal bowel movements, then constipation, normal bowel, constipation, in what is usually a random and unpredictable cycle, this may last for a few months or even years.

Some people seem to go straight from normal bowel to loose bowel very quickly and don't get constipation.

These scenarios are usually associated with some stomach discomfort, anyone diagnosed medically with these type of bowel problems over a number of years, are usually said to have "irritable bowel syndrome", IBS.

Its when your digestive tract suddenly flips into a state of permanent loose bowels and stays in the loose bowel condition, and the walls of your digestive tract open up that we have a serious problem, this is where I define the difference between I.B.S and the emergency state, its when this permanent loose bowel state of affairs exists that we begin to feel tired and weak all the time, and many of the classic and advanced intolerance symptoms begin to develop, its now that chronic fatigue or M.E begins to take hold of you.

So in the early years our digestive system is initially able to cope with this sequence of events, and the intolerance foods, then we begin to produce less bile and pancreatic enzymes, our ability to break down these foods is impaired, and our ability to detoxify is also impaired.

Initially you won't realise that you are slightly bloated, and you won't feel tired. Then in many of us, our digestive tract slows the food through our system, as described above, the underlying cause is due to the lack of bile and enzyme production, this often gives us constipation for a short period at some stage in the development of food intolerance.

This is nature at work, its slowing things down (the peristalsis, the snake action) and trying desperately to extract the nutrients from what we are eating. But it can only slow our peristalsis down to a certain point, if your digestive tract came to a stop, you would die.

At this point you feel relatively ok and have energy and are not tired all the time. Many people seem to hover around this stage, and switch between loose bowels and constipation for many years; you may have loose bowels and constipation on the same day.

As I said before it's at about this point, where we often switch into permanent loose bowel, and that is where I define the difference between irritable bowel syndrome (IBS), and the emergency state.

It's at about this point that Helicobacter Pylori can raise its head and begin to cause a problem.

Helicobacter Pylori is a bacterium that can live in your stomach, and cause irritation of the stomach lining. In many people who are healthy this bacteria causes no problem, but for people like us with food intolerance, it can cause stomach discomfort, and even ulcers, when coupled with an inability to break down food.

THE EMERGING EMERGENCY STATE

In the advanced stages of food intolerance, you will have a diminished ability to break down food, even if peristalsis slows right down, peristalsis (the snake action) cannot stop, so it will have to change the way it functions, and speed up.

If you are producing very little bile, enzymes, and hormones from your liver and pancreas, your digestive tract will have no option but to speed up your peristalsis permanently, giving you permanent loose bowels.

So the digestive tract will be flipped into permanent loose bowels. We have now just slipped into the more advanced stages of intolerance, "The emergency state", and compensation.

Now instead of the digestive tract slowly filtering the nutrients into our body, it opens the walls of our digestive systems, and speeds the flow of food through our digestive tract, by revving up the peristalsis throughout the digestive tract, this is natures way of trying to expel the intolerance foods, but continue to try and extract some nutrients from what we are eating.

The underlying cause is due to the lack of bile enzyme and hormone production, from the liver and pancreas, undigested food will be washed through the digestive tract, and some of the good nutrients are being treated as toxins along with the actual toxins.

At this point some people develop the late onset Celiac condition, with flattened villi and antibody reaction, these people absorb very little and loose weight.

If you think you are in this category you may be advised to have a blood test for Celiac disease, but you must realise that if you are a late onset celiac, then it is most likely that you have a clogged liver or gallstones, this is the underlying cause of your celiac condition, and a series of gallbladder and liver flushes are required.

Other people begin to bloat in appearance, (retention) this is the usual reaction to gained intolerance without the Celiac scenario and the one most of us have.

Now we have a serious problem, in that the mixtures wrong in our bowel, and some of the nutrients are able to fall through the gut wall in the wrong concentrations, some of the nutrients do not appear to be absorbed at all, or at least very little. This scenario is often called leaky gut syndrome.

This is going to make you feel ill and very tired, but at least nature's way is keeping you alive.

If you stay in this state for any period of time, your digestive tract and bodily organs will deteriorate, and eventually there is the possibility that other problems, could or will develop in your body, your immune system will weaken, your lymphatic system will become sluggish, you will feel stiff and

ache. All this will leave you much less resistant to viruses and more susceptible to illnesses.
There is a strong possibility that in advanced cases, you will develop digestive tract problems, such as ulcerative colitis, crohns disease, diverticulitis, gastric or duodenal ulcers, colonitis, and many other conditions, even bowel cancer.

SCENARIOS

So, we have many scenarios here, including Irritable Bowel (I.B.S), Celiac (wheat gluten intolerance), and wheat dairy intolerance, eventually leading to the more extreme and more advanced emergency state.

These three conditions almost certainly have the same causal factor, too much wheat, sugar, and dairy products, or more to the point processed fortified, high protein wheat products, processed raw sugar, and too many pasteurised dairy products, causing clogging of the liver.

CELIAC DISEASE

People with celiac disease have flattened villi (protrusions in their duodenum and jejunum) and produce antibodies against the gluten in the wheat. With this condition the digestive tract becomes seriously impaired, because the villi are flattened the absorptive surface area is much less, and also acts like a mat, blocking other nutrient absorption pathways within the lining of the digestive tract, therefore you are less able to break down, and absorb the foods that you eat, especially in their duodenum and jejunum, and therefore in the advanced stages they loose weight rapidly, and feel very weak and tired.

These people will have loose bowels, and a speeded up peristalsis. In this state a vicious circle ensues, bile and enzymes production begins to degrade and reduce, and the digestive tract becomes far less permeable, therefore fewer and fewer elements are absorbed, causing bile and enzyme production to degrade and reduce even further. If this condition is not diagnosed early enough, failure of vital organs can occur.

It is said that people with this condition can never eat wheat based products ever again, even a trace of gluten affects them, although strangely, they can sometimes eat oats, which contain a very similar gluten protein to wheat.

People with this condition usually have a clogged liver, and impaired pancreatic and kidney function.

Many Celiacs have gallstones, and if they flush their gallbladder and liver, they often find that they can then eat small amounts of wheat, dairy, and sugar again with no reaction.

Indeed many Celiacs have had their gallbladder removed; and they are still celiac, but if they flush their liver out, and get it clean again, they too can begin to tolerate small amounts of wheat, dairy and sugar, this only adds weight to the argument that many diagnosed celiacs are not true celiacs, all they had was a clogged liver, this gave them their wheat and dairy intolerance, and caused their villi to flatten.

IRRITABLE BOWEL SYNDROME

People with irritable bowel (IBS) don't necessarily have the walls of their digestive tract porous all the time (leaky gut syndrome), they don't get the celiac symptoms of flattened villi, and therefore don't always get intensely tired, don't necessarily feel too ill, and don't get many of the symptoms in the list on pages 18 to 21. However, they can have a speeded up peristalsis, but not necessarily all the time. They seem to stop on the edge of the precipice of either, celiac disease, or the food intolerance induced "emergency state".

Many people diagnosed with I.B.S, have often advanced further into food intolerance since their diagnosis, and by the time I see them they are often in the "emergency state", with permanent loose bowels, and digestive compensation, unless they have changed their diet somewhat, which is often the case, because they have realised that eating less wheat and dairy improved their condition, in which case they have often arrested their symptoms, but not recovered their ability to break down these foods.

Therefore they often have many of the advanced symptoms of intolerance, and have a high score when they add up the points in the symptoms list on page 20.

This condition is also associated with a clogged liver and impaired pancreatic and kidney function. A series of gallbladder and liver flushes will definitely be required for full recovery to take place.

THE EMERGENCY STATE

The emergency state describes people who are not celiac, but have a reaction to gluten or wheat, but don't get flattened villi in their digestive tract.

People with this condition have a permanent speeded up peristalsis, and are often in digestive compensation stage 3, the "emergency state" and have very loose bowels, and the wall of their digestive tract is far more open and porous (leaky gut syndrome) than what would be considered normal, allowing some nutrients to fall through the intestine wall into the bloodstream in the wrong concentrations or form.

Some nutrients are not broken down, synthesised or absorbed, this makes you feel ill, weak, tired etc.
Although with this condition you don't loose weight, but bloat, and every molecule of your body seems to expand, its not fat, its retention of fluids, you look like michelin man, rounded rather than fat, this is partly due to the lack of nutrient absorption.

When you first adopt the recovery diet, and begin to recover you don't only loose weight, but seem to shrink as well, you usually pass lots of water for about a month, this would indicate that you have had some measure of water retention.

You could almost say that it's the opposite to celiac disease, in that the villi are not flattened, and you don't produce antibodies, but the walls of your digestive tract are very open causing an over absorption of some nutrients and under absorption of others. It appears that late onset celiac disease, and "the emergency state" have similar causal factors, wheat, dairy and sugar consumption over a lifetime, clogging the gallbladder and liver

This is the category I fell into, and if you have most of the symptoms on pages 18 to 21, then there is a strong possibility that you too are in this category, especially if any tests for celiac disease came back negative.

People with this condition can be just as intolerant to wheat or oats as a celiac, and have many of the same symptoms, many people who are intolerant to wheat without the celiac criteria, of flattened villi and antibodies, are also very sensitive to oats, both conditions have the same causal factor with dramatically different digestive tract reactions, this is what divides a celiac from someone who is in the "emergency state".

People with this condition almost certainly have a clogged liver, and possibly kidney and/ or gallstones, yeast overgrowth, and impaired pancreatic and kidney function. Therefore the gallbladder and liver flushes, and kidney cleanses will have to be undertaken, to gain full recovery.

OBSERVATIONS

So, as you can see there are subtle differences between these three conditions, celiac disease, I.B.S, and the "emergency state" of the bowel, although the causal factors are very similar, or could be said to be the same.

I was able to track the food through my digestive system using the reactions chart on pages 30-31, and found the worst affected parts of the digestive tract seem to be the duodenum, jejunum and the latter sections of the large intestine where food passes from the colon to the rectum, and fluids are re cycled.

In early recovery you should go to the toilet as soon as you feel like it, if you don't go to the toilet as soon as you feel like you should, you will begin to feel slightly ill, as some of the fluids that are being reabsorbed at this point seem to carry with them unwanted elements, and toxic wastes, and swamp your ability to filter them, and detoxify them.

This is due to the reduced ability of the organs related to detoxification, such as the liver and kidneys.

This is an extremely important reason why people such as us, should stay away from anything that produces toxins, or foods that are difficult to break down, such as wheat and dairy products, or anything directly toxic such as alcohol, our systems have lost the ability to cope with large amounts of processed food and toxins.

We start to develop many of the symptoms in the list of symptoms on pages 18 to 21.

The main problem is that you will feel very tired, this is natures way of trying to repair your system, after all if nature puts you to sleep your body has time to begin repairs.

While you are asleep you are not going to ingest any of the intolerance foods that your digestive tract has desperately been trying to cope with for such a long time.

Now if you keep ingesting the intolerance foods whilst any of these conditions exist, your digestive tract cannot repair itself, you are slowly going to get worse and worse, and degrade and clog up your liver, impair your kidneys, and pancreatic function, this will impede your ability to produce bile and enzymes and detoxify even further.

The thyroid gland can also be affected, I often find that intolerants have been diagnosed with thyroid problems, and are taking thyroxin to try and redress the problem, this is alleviating symptoms and not addressing the cause or causes of their condition, if they are given the recovery regime in this book their condition improves by leaps and bounds, they are often food intolerants, with the pre described scenarios, and often recovery of their digestive tract reduces dramatically their need for large doses of thyroxin.

Although I have to say that if thyroxin has been taken for a lengthy period of time, the thyroid gland appears to stop producing any thyroxin at all, these people are then reliant on thyroxin for the rest of their lives.

If you do not follow the recovery programme you will become more and more tired and weak in little time, and in the case of the emergency state will have to eat vast amounts of food to keep functioning, because you're not absorbing it properly.

However, what you do absorb in the case of the emergency state will mainly be carbohydrate, and the lack of some vital nutrients such as fats, proteins, vitamins and minerals, will lead to retention and give you a bloated appearance in your face and body, (the Michelin man effect), as apposed to celiac disease where you will stop absorbing many elements and will loose weight over a period of time.

The exception to this seems to be irritable bowel syndrome (IBS), where people switch between loose bowels and constipation, these people seem to stay in this condition without sliding any further, and don't disappear into the mire of the emergency state, with permanent loose bowels, and don't develop celiac disease.

The common factor in all these scenarios is too much processed wheat, sugar and dairy products, ingested over a lifetime, at too high a concentration. Look in your shopping basket and see how many products contain wheat, sugar and dairy products, this is all high protein and carbohydrate. Wheat dairy and sugar are in many foods you wouldn't expect them to be found in.

The problem with the true celiac condition, is that you will be producing antibodies against the gluten in the wheat, and this may or will stay with you all your life, so anything containing gluten may have to be avoided for life, although I have to say that many celiacs are not celiacs, all they have is food intolerance and an inability to break down food, due to a clogged liver.

M.E, YUPPIE FLU

I have found that many people who claim to have recovered from ME or yuppie flu, often they have not fully recovered, they have subconsciously and actually learnt that they react to wheat and dairy products, and they have learnt to eat far less of these products, and subsequently they feel much better.

They have however not fully recovered, but have learnt to live with their condition, and are necessarily subconsciously controlling it by limiting what they eat, mainly in relation to wheat and dairy products.

These people have very often been wrongly diagnosed, and in reality many of them have actually gained food intolerance, and have a clogged liver, this is the cause of their problems, and not the pigeonhole diagnosis of M.E, which they have been allotted.

THE CRUCIAL KEY TO RECOVERY

Where food intolerance is concerned by far the most important area of the human anatomy involves the liver, pancreas and common bile duct.

If there is any restriction, impairment, clogging, coagulation, or resistance to the free production and flow of bile from the liver, and down through the entire common bile duct, then the digestive tract cannot function properly, thus malabsorption will occur and the whole of your body will suffer as a consequence.

I cannot over emphasise the importance of regaining the ability to break down and absorb properly the foods you eat. It's absolutely crucial, essential, vital, and critical, that you have or regain this free flow of bile enzymes and hormones down the common bile duct.

This can only be achieved by making absolutely certain that your liver and gallbladder are clean, then and only then will you have a free and uninterrupted, unimpeded production and flow of bile enzymes and hormones to break down your food.

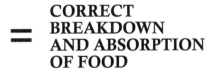

FREEFLOW OF BILE ENZIMES AND HORMONES DOWN THE COMMON BILE DUCT = CORRECT BREAKDOWN AND ABSORPTION OF FOOD

We can only achieve this essential situation by flushing out the liver and gallbladder with the liver and gallbladder flush, as detailed, on page 238, and cleaning the kidneys with the beetroot cleanse as detailed on page 223, and the herbal cleanse as detailed on page 224.

DIGESTIVE TRACT TIMING AND I.B.S

This can be quite a complicated subject, it mainly revolves around peristalsis, this is the muscle wave action that carries food through the entire digestive tract, this wave action is similar to the way a snake takes food along its body, when it swallows food you can see it travelling along its body, this is a graphic example of muscle wave action at work.

Correct timing is essential within the digestive tract, especially in the relationship between the liver, common bile duct and the duodenum.

Any restriction in the free flow of bile down the common bile duct will affect this peristaltic muscle wave action and will influence directly the way your digestive tract will perform or react to the ingestion of different types of food.

So, lets look firstly at how the digestive tract functions when it is fit and healthy.

Food is chewed in the mouth where saliva mixes with the food, this is the first step in braking down the food you eat, the food then travels down the oesophagus into the stomach where the stomach secretes acid from the stomach wall, the food then passes into the duodenum where bile enzymes and hormones flood in down the common bile duct to mix with the food and further aid in breaking it down, the food then passes through the entire length of the digestive tract where all the nutrients are extracted from it, at different points on its journey through the intestine.

In a stable and normal digestive tract the food is carried through the digestive tract by the muscle wave action called peristalsis, in a normal environment this wave action is regular and within a stable band, food is carried through the entire digestive tract at a regulated speed, by far the most important part of this controlled and regulated movement of food, is the transition and speed at which it flows through the duodenum, and past the common bile duct.

In normal circumstances a free flow of bile enzymes and hormones is able to travel unimpeded down the common bile duct and mix with the food, therefore a stable peristalsis can be attained, there is no reason for the digestive tract to change the speed that the food is moved through the digestive tract, therefore a healthy state of affairs can be observed, food will be effectively broken down, and all the elements the body requires will be absorbed and utilized to run your bodily functions very efficiently.

Now lets look at what begins to happen when you become intolerant to wheat and or dairy products.
You have H.D.L, L.D.L and V.L.D.L (high density, ,low density and very low density lipoprotein) in your blood.

If you eat too much wheat protein, dairy products and processed carbohydrate (sugar) you will distort these molecules, these molecules are basically the cholesterol in your blood, your liver needs to see these molecules because your liver produces cholesterol, if these molecules are thickened or swollen or distorted your liver cannot detect many of them, they cannot get through the membranes into your liver cells, so your liver assumes that you have low cholesterol, and begins to produce copious amounts of cholesterol.

Some of this cholesterol begins to coagulate within the liver and begins to clog the liver and eventually cause gallstones to develop, this leads to the liver becoming less efficient and producing less bile, this impinges on the pancreas and it too begins to loose its performance, and therefore less enzymes and hormones are produced.

If your gallbladder is much larger than normal, because it is full of gallstones, it can also push against, and partially flatten and restrict the part of your digestive tract that runs behind your gallbladder, this is unusual but it can cause a restriction in your digestive tract and compound the problems we are about to discuss.

Bearing these scenarios in mind, we can now begin to look at what happens when you begin to gain intolerance to some foods, usually wheat and or dairy products, food is chewed as normal and mixed with saliva in your mouth, it then moves down your oesophagus into your stomach, this is where the first problems begin to occur.

Because of the coagulation and clogging within the liver you are not producing and freely passing enough bile enzymes or hormones to break down your food, your digestive tract knows within twenty minutes of the food being in your stomach, whether it can produce enough bile enzymes and hormones to break down the food you have eaten, when it transgresses into your digestive tract.

If it knows it cannot produce enough bile enzymes and hormones your digestive tract will then begin to compensate, by producing more stomach acid, your body is very clever and has evolved to do this, it does this to help, and aid your digestive tract extract nutrients from the food you are eating, it's trying to break your food down within your stomach, far more than would be considered the norm, and before your food gets to your intestine, your extremely clever body and digestive tract have evolved over millions of years to do this trick, to keep you alive as long as possible if you are losing the ability to extract nutrients within the intestine.

The side effect of this is to give you acid reflux and indigestion.

Now the food you ate maybe 3 hours ago passes into the duodenum, where we encounter the next and most important and major problem.

Remember peristalsis the muscle wave action that carries food through your digestive tract, it now begins to change in the way it functions, due to your liver being clogged and having gallstones.

Because of the previously mentioned over production of cholesterol due to your diet, causing distorted HDL, LDL, and VLDL, your liver becomes sluggish and this impinges on your pancreas, you then produce less of the vital bile, enzymes, and hormones required to break down food.

This decreased amount of bile, enzymes, and hormones flows down the common bile duct into the duodenum, and mixes with the food you ate 3 hours ago; these elements are vital to break down this food.

You only have one chance to get enough bile enzymes and hormones into your food as it passes the common bile duct; your common bile duct enters into the first part of your duodenum, just after your stomach.

If you have eaten something which is difficult to break down, such as bread or dairy products you will need lots of bile, enzymes, and hormones to break them down efficiently, if the situation begins to develop where there is not enough bile enzymes or hormones available then obviously you will not break down your food properly.

Again your body is very clever and begins to "compensate" by initially slowing down the peristalsis, as well as producing copious amounts of stomach acid, as discussed previously, the peristalsis will slow down the food as it passes the common bile duct, to try and allow more time for the reduced flow of bile enzymes and hormones to get into the food you ate.

This state of affairs will give you constipation because the peristalsis may slow down to a crawl to try and buy more time to get those vital hormones bile and enzymes into your food. These scenarios happen in the earlier stages of intolerance and lead to constipation.

Now we will move on to the next stage of digestive compensation in the more advanced cases of food intolerance.

We now have an even bigger problem looming, your peristalsis cannot stop or your digestive tract would stop all together, and you would die.

So again your body is very clever, as you begin to produce even less bile, enzymes, and hormones your peristalsis will arrive at a point, if you have eaten something very difficult to break down, where it will suddenly speed up, because it knows, or more to the point, your digestive tract has worked out within twenty minutes of ingesting food, whether it cannot possibly produce and pass enough bile, enzymes, and hormones into the food you have eaten, to break it down, however slowly the peristalsis goes, remember the peristalsis cannot stop.

We now have a big problem, the only thing your peristalsis can do is speed up, patently we are going to have very little bile enzymes and hormones in the food we have eaten, because of the speed that this food is passing through the digestive tract, and more importantly how fast the food is passing through the duodenum and passing the common bile duct due to the revved up peristalsis.

Now we will have loose bowels.

But how are you going to extract some nutrients from the food you have eaten, there is going to be very little bile enzymes and hormones in your food?

So to try and extract some nutrients form the food in your digestive tract, the walls of your intestine will become much more porous and allow nutrient molecules to fall through the gut wall in sizes larger than would be considered normal. This is when you begin to feel tired, because the mixtures wrong in your blood, but at least your body is getting enough nutrients to stay alive.

So you have gained food intolerance through lack of bile enzyme and hormone production, and more importantly the lack of free flow of bile enzymes and hormones down the common bile duct, due to the clogging of the liver and gallstones.

Lets assume that your have become very intolerant, and have all the previously discussed problems within your digestive tract.

Now lets say for arguments sake you ate a salad, something that is very easy to break down, your peristalsis will slow right down, because your body knows it can break down a salad, its producing just enough bile enzymes and hormones to cope with breaking down the salad, although your digestive tract will have to slow your peristalsis right down making you constipated.

Now lets take another scenario, and argue that you have eaten something which is difficult to break down, wheat or dairy products, steak pie and chips, your body and digestive tract knows it cannot produce or pass freely enough bile, enzymes, or hormones to break these products down, the peristalsis speeds up, opening the gut wall and making it more porous, and giving you loose bowels.

Do these scenarios ring any bells with you; well they should, because I have just described what is known as IBS, "Irritable bowel syndrome".

Some people go so far into this state of affairs that they have a speeded up peristalsis permanently, this I refer to as the "emergency state", as described previously in this chapter.

Others develop flattened villi, and gain late onset celiac disease also described earlier in this chapter, celiacs absorb very little of the food they have eaten, and often begin to loose weight, and feel very weak and tired all the time.

So as you can see its all about bile and enzyme production, if there isn't enough time for sufficient amounts of bile enzymes and hormones to mix with your food in the duodenum, in the correct amount to break the foods down, then the peristalsis and digestive tract will respond in the appropriate manner, by either speeding up, or slowing down the peristalsis, and making the digestive tract more, or less porous.

The only way to remedy this situation is to adopt the advised diet in this book, and flush the gallbladder and liver and recover the kidneys, so that you produce a free unimpeded unrestricted flow, with copious amounts of bile enzymes and hormones flooding down the common bile duct, to break down whatever food is in the duodenum.

When, and only when this state of affairs exists can the peristalsis stabilise, and stay within its stable band whatever food is ingested.

I know this concept may take a little time to grasp, but once you understand the importance of the scenarios I have just described, you will understand the imperative of making sure you have a free flow of bile, enzymes, and hormones, this obviously involves the cleansing of the liver, refer to the gallbladder and liver flush chapter for, details of the flush see page 228.

There is a more detailed description of digestive function beginning on page 248, where digestive inability is discussed in far more detail.

THE LIVER AND GALLSTONES

THE SYMPTOMS OF GALLSTONES

- Aching and stiffness in one or other or both shoulders, usually right shoulders.

- Hypoglycaemia (low blood sugar) in extreme cases.

- Pain just under your right lower rib cage and running round and into your back.

- You may also have an ache just under your right shoulder blade, especially after sleeping, this is only in advanced cases.

- Slight pain two or three inches down from your lower right ribcage (often with I.B.S)

- Jaundice (yellowy appearance of skin, and the whites of your eyes)

- Oily skin, especially around bridge of nose and forehead.

- General lethargy.

- Tan in sun very easily and readily.

- Fluey sinuses, slight nasal cold.

- Light coloured stools, or light then dark stools, (very good indicator of clogged liver)

- Slight nausea after eating fatty or oily foods.

- Pain half hour after eating fatty or oily food.

- Splitting of the bottom lip.

- Dry cracking skin at corners of mouth.

- Ulcers on or inside the bottom lip, in advanced cases.

- Dry bottom lip.

- Candida

- Yeast overgrowth

- Lost sense of thirst, (in extreme cases)

- Lines running the length of your fingernails.

• Itching all over, not all the time but on regular occasions.

• Chest pains around your chest area, random pains around your chest area, in advanced cases. (If you are experiencing a tight chest, like your chest is being sat on, and this is accompanied by pains in your arms, especially left arm, please consult your doctor immediately)

In the early stages of formation, gallstones will not give you any obvious symptoms, but they will slowly be inhibiting the free flow of bile down the common bile duct.

Whether the gallstones are in your liver, or gallbladder dictates the level of impaired free flow of bile, often the trigger to moving gallstones into a position where they cause definite and noticeable symptoms is violent exercise, such as squat thrusts in particular, or a violent event like a bad fall or an accident, this can jolt the liver area and cause gallstones to move, if they collect in the wrong place they can suddenly impair the free flow of bile very quickly, and symptoms can begin to develop in as little as a week after the event.

There is a very strong possibility you may have gallstones after years of food intolerance, this is a very common occurrence and usually the case.

In fact I would go so far as to say that it is unlikely that you don't have gallstones after years of eating the wrong foods, and the standard western diet. Gallstones impair the production and flow of bile.

Even if you don't have gallstones a gallbladder and liver flush is recommended, to clean out any chaff, or the early formation of crystals, which lead to gallstones.

If you have many gallstones they could partially block your bile ducts, and cause aching or pain in your lower right ribcage and possibly under your right shoulder blade.

If you only have slightly raised cholesterol levels there is a very strong possibility you will have gallstones and a flush is strongly recommended, people with very high cholesterol levels, don't tend to make many gallstones, as I will explain later in this chapter.

Before I begin to describe what happens to cause you to have raised cholesterol and/or gallstones, bear in mind that the liver produces cholesterol and that gallstones in the main are made of cholesterol.

The gluten content of bread is the protein element, and a very highly concentrated protein; too much protein linked with sugar and dairy product intake, can cause gallstones and a clogged liver.

Excessive protein, dairy products and processed carbohydrate (sugar) consumption leads to thickening or swelling of the blood vessels base membranes, this prevents some of the cholesterol LDL (LDL=low density lipoprotein) and VLDL (VLDL=very low density lipoprotein) in the blood from entering the liver cells, then the liver assumes that there must be a shortage of HDL, LDL and VLDL in the blood, and the liver begins to produce more cholesterol.

This adds to the cholesterol already in the blood, which the liver did not detect, and a vicious circle ensues, and an excessive build up of cholesterol in the blood.

This excess production of cholesterol laden bile from the liver can lead initially to clogging within the liver, and eventually to gallstones.

Gallstones originate in the liver and then migrate to the gallbladder and continue to gather cholesterol and enlarge.

Importantly people who have high cholesterol in their blood, often do not tend to make many gallstones, and therefore rarely tend to gain full blown intolerance to food.

This is because they don't tend to coagulate cholesterol within the liver and begin to make large cholesterol type gallstones, the excess cholesterol in these people passes more freely into their digestive tract, but if they are on a bad diet, their digestive tract is more porous than it should be, and some of this cholesterol is re absorbed, and adds to the cholesterol in the blood, which the liver could not see, therefore they have very high blood cholesterol levels.

If the diet in this book is adopted fully, the blood cholesterol levels in these people will begin to stabilise, its not the fat causing the problem, ingested fat is just adding to the cholesterol problem, it's the excess consumption of wheat gluten, dairy and sugar that is the underlying cause of their problems, distorting their HDL, LDL, and VLDL.

Those of us who are susceptible, and gain intolerance to food, tend to coagulate the cholesterol within the liver and gallbladder, and form gallstones, rather than pass it into the blood, and we therefore form cholesterol type gallstones, those of us in this category don't tend to have excessively raised cholesterol, often serum levels only reach about 4.8 to 5.

The detection of gallstones is usually done by an ultrasound scan of the gallbladder, but this does not always show up the gallstones. I have found many people who have had an ultrasound scan, and have been told, "you definitely do not have gallstones" but after following their symptoms for a while, I was sure they had gallstones, and after some persuasion they did a gallbladder and liver flush, or a series of gallbladder and liver flushes, and low and behold, they passed hundreds of gallstones. And after many flushes, they cleaned their liver of stones and chaff, and their stomach discomfort, and food intolerance symptoms, went away.

So, if you've had a scan for gallstones don't take it as gospel that you don't have any.

Many people have gallstones and no pain at all, but after experimenting with people that have gallstones and no symptoms at all, i have found that they definitely break down and absorb foods much better after a gallbladder and liver flush, or as many flushes as are necessary to clean out the liver, and gallbladder, they then find they have to eat less or they put on weight more readily, although they tell me they can control their weight very easily because they are not constantly hungry.

Many Celiacs and people with M.E have had their gallbladders removed, this is done without realising, that the gallstones have formed as a consequence of a lifetime of over indulgence, in high gluten protein products, wheat, dairy and refined sugar, and their digestive problems, and tiredness or exhaustion are the end result.

But its no good just removing the gallbladder, although they shouldn't have removed it in the first place, unless it was perforated, infected or calcified, you must also flush out the forming stones and chaff in the liver, this is why these people very often do not recover properly, and are often told when they have returning symptoms, you are having a phantom gallstone attack, or you may be told that you have developed I.B.S.

There is no phantom, it's the chaff or sludge left in the liver moving through the ducts in the liver and welling up in the ducting, causing pain and the many scenarios leading to continued intolerance to food. If you are one of these people then a gallbladder and liver flush or flushes is essential for full recovery to take place, even though you have had your gallbladder removed.

If you have had your gallbladder removed, you must leave 12 months or so for your system to heal properly, before you attempt a liver and gallbladder flush.

I have also found, and people who have flushed their liver often report, that they do not feel as hungry, this is due to the fact that they are breaking down synthesising and absorbing all the elements in their food far more efficiently, and their mind is subconsciously telling them that their body has all the elements to run at its optimum, and switches off all the hunger pangs. Therefore a healthy diet is easier to follow, without feeling hungry all the time.

Another noticeable improvement is in relation to yeast overgrowth. If you flush your liver then the yeast overgrowth dies back much faster, this is due to the fact that your liver is producing better quality bile, your pancreas will be working more efficiently, and therefore your breakdown and absorption of food is much better, and therefore the gut flora is better balanced, and the conditions for the yeast overgrowth to thrive are very much reduced and eventually eradicated completely.

The liver is a vital part of your digestive system, it's the filter and detoxification plant of your body along with the kidneys. It's like an I.C.I chemicals plant with thousands of pipes, tubes, filters, storage facilities and production systems, only millions of times more complicated. You only have one of them so you need to respect it.

When it's working at its optimum it has an amazing ability to filter out toxins from your body, it produces up to three pints of bile a day to help break down foods, it synthesises thousands of elements every minute, stores minerals and vitamins, produces hormones, and interacts these elements in a myriad of complex processes, to aid in the breakdown and absorption of foods in the digestive tract, and also helps to balance and control toxins.

All the evidence is now pointing to the fact that we could have been clogging our livers even as babies.

If you were fed cows milk rather than breast-fed as a baby, and then weaned onto solids with wheat based products, then there is a very strong possibility that your liver had begun to clog up even in your very young years, and a possibility that those of us who are susceptible to the long term over ingestion of wheat, dairy and processed sugar, could even have developed gallstone, and clogging of the liver, as young as two to five years of age, although there would be very few obvious symptoms at this young age.

If the liver begins to degrade or clog up through years of eating the wrong foods, mainly high wheat protein, dairy and processed sugar, then you're not going to detoxify properly or produce enough quality bile.

The lack of filtration and detoxification, and the impaired ability to break down absorb and interact foods, will leave you feeling tired and ill, and many symptoms will begin to emerge such as those listed in the symptoms chapter on pages 18 to 21.

Luckily, nature and millions of years of evolution, have developed a liver that is capable of taking a lot of punishment, and still function although in a decreased capacity, however it is capable of rebuilding itself if the correct diet is adopted although a series of gallbladder and liver flushes will be necessary, to clean out the liver properly.

Then and only then will you produce more bile enzymes and hormones, and quality bile enzymes and hormones, and remember the pancreas is also affected if the liver has been impaired, this will also begin to recover, and then the chain of events involved in breaking down, and absorbing foods, will be much improved.

This in turn helps cell regeneration, and conversion of proteins and carbohydrates, and will help to sustain and repair other organs such as the pancreas, spleen, and kidneys.

The detoxification side of your liver is an extremely complex problem, involving lots of interactive processes in the digestive tract, and at a molecular level. Your liver is one of the component parts in a complex chain of events when it comes to detoxification, involving interactions of different vitamins, minerals, enzymes, and many other elements, and many other organs of the body. So to get detoxification going again is a much more difficult task, mainly involving your diet, this is yet another reason why the diet is so important in recovery.

Even good natural foods contain toxic elements, but the liver easily deals with these natural foods so overload does not occur. But in those of us who have gained intolerance, the digestive tract is not breaking down, and synthesising foods and elements properly, and the mixtures wrong, so some of the good nutrients are treated as toxins as well as the actual toxins.

This overwhelms your ability to detoxify, and your liver along with other organs is slowly overloaded, and will begin to clog up enlarge and degrade.

It can filter up to 1 litre of blood per minute, so any congestion seriously impedes filtration and blood flow and seriously affects bile, cholesterol, enzyme, hormones and protein production, conversion filtration and elimination of toxins is also impeded, and the lymphatic system is overloaded and unable to discard dead cells efficiently.

This in turn leads to the degradation and enlargement of other organs, especially the stomach, spleen, small and large intestines, pancreas, thyroid and gallbladder, thus putting pressure on the heart. Blood flow to extremities of the body is also impaired.

This is why so many people who have intolerance report dead limbs when sleeping, or tingling in hands and feet.

A catastrophic chain of events can ensue, and if not checked, even liver or other organ failure could be the end result, or at the very least permanent liver damage, so its vital that you make sure your liver is cleaned and flushed out properly.

The previous is describing what's happening in very simple terms, if I went into the detail you would only get bored, and probably not understand it anyway, so I will leave it at that. Unless I'm being presumptuous, in which case I apologise.

If you wanted to put the perfect recipe together for gallstones or a clogged up liver, then the following would be the ultimate scenario.

Eat too much so called processed, fast pre packed or junk foods every day, eat too much bread, drink too much alcohol and smoke, drink too much tea, or coffee, eat too many high wheat based protein foods, drink too many soft drinks, eat too much processed sugar, consume too many dairy products, don't eat fruit and lots of vegetables, and don't exercise.

If this is you, which it probably is or was, along with 90% of the population, then your liver and kidneys will have to work like lunatics every day, to break down what you are eating, and more to the point detoxify your system.

You are ingesting or inhaling thousands of toxins, your liver along with other organs have to detoxify these toxins, and in a desperate, and unbelievably complex process of interaction, try to keep a balance in your system. Understandably eventually your liver says, I've had enough of this, I'm going on a go slow, if it makes him ill I don't care any more, I can only work so hard.

If you work too hard you get tired, so does your liver.

Failures in the liver impact on every organ in the body, and these will degrade along with the liver, especially vital organs like the pancreas, and kidneys.

It's like running your car with the choke out, it will keep chugging along, but it's running very inefficiently, with far too much fuel, it will be weak and sluggish just as you are.

So we have to begin by eating low toxin, high detoxification foods, with good natural vitamin and mineral elements, to make life as easy as we can for your liver, then it can put its feet up now and then, and begin to repair itself after years or even decades of brutal punishment.

You should use milk thistle to help clean your liver in the early stages of recovery, this will make your urine very yellow at first, as the toxins are released, and after a week or two your urine will return to normal, this is a good sign that you have expelled some toxins and made one of the first steps in cleaning out the liver.

Although as I have said before a series of gallbladder and liver flushes are vital to flush the liver. Even after you have flushed out the liver, with the gallbladder and liver flush or flushes, and adopted the correct diet, the liver will take about 6 months to recover properly, and then a further two years for other organs to repair themselves.

There is no magic cure, it's a case of adopting in general a new lifestyle in your eating and drinking habits, this does not mean that you can't ever drink alcohol again, or eat some of the more harmful foods, but be aware of the long term consequences of over indulgence of these products, after all that's how you got into this condition in the first place!

THE PANCREAS

The pancreas is a vital component in the breakdown and absorpsion of foods, it produces lots of enzymes and hormones, which interact with bile from the liver to break down foods, and also control blood sugar levels.

If this organ is damaged it can have dire consequences for your digestive tract, impairing the production of enzymes and hormones, and thus the breakdown and absorption of food.

One of the major factors in pancreas and liver damage today is alcohol, and binge drinking. If you go out and binge drink, lets say you drink 7 bottles of strong beer or 7 pints of beer, it will leave you noticeably weak and slightly tired for two or three days, even if you are fit and healthy.

If you have food intolerance then it will make you feel unwell for up to a week, this is because your enzyme and hormone production has been affected, and many toxins have been produced, food is not broken down synthesised or absorbed properly, and going back to the liver, the liver is overwhelmed by the toxins, no wonder you feel weak tired and!!

If you go out binge drinking, it will take about ten days for your pancreas to recover to the point it was at before you had the drink. So if you binge drink once a week, you are slowly degrading and probably damaging or at least degrading your pancreas, along with the liver, because your pancreas and liver will never have the chance to recover properly.

Again if you eat too much junk, fast or highly processed high protein and in particular refined carbohydrate foods (sugars), your pancreas has to work like a lunatic to produce the enzymes and hormones necessary to break down and regulate these foods.

It is particularly susceptible to concentrated substances so often found in modern fast foods. Think of the E numbers and artificial sweeteners, preservatives, and flavourings. Read any label on a pre packed, ready to eat food and/or drink, and they will contain many of these elements.

Aspartame a sweetener found in many slimming products and soft drinks is very toxic if ingested in large quantities, and an increasing amount of evidence is building which makes frightening reading in relation to this sweetener, and the devastating effect it can have on many organs of the body, if ingested over a long period of time, when Aspartame interacts with some chemicals in your body it converts to formaldehyde, formaldehyde is used to embalm bodies, so it stands to reason that this not only damages the pancreas but many other organs as well, and the toxic aspartame is extremely difficult for the body to expel.

To add to this the modern diet contains too much protein and sugar, mainly wheat protein and raw sugar, all of this leads to the overloading and degradation of the pancreas, leaving us less able to break down synthesise and absorb foods, so your digestive tract degrades even more, leading us down the chain of events so often mentioned in this book which lead to food intolerance. Correct enzyme and hormone production is absolutely essential for the break down and absorption of food.

This is why some pancreatic conditions such as diabetes are becoming more common, or should I say reaching epidemic proportions.

Basically the pancreas will loose the ability to produce enzymes, insulin and hormones, which are responsible for efficient breakdown of food, and the regulating blood sugar levels.

The consequential upset in gut flora, and the malabsorption, will lead to gallstones and a clogged liver, initially this overloads the pancreas even more and often if the liver is not functioning properly, its left to the pancreas to do most of the work in trying to break down foods, and regulate an increasing excess of blood glucose levels.

Once you begin to loose the ability to break down oils, fats and proteins, you need to understand that your body will be living in the main off sugar (glucose) for energy, so your pancreas will have to work overtime producing more insulin every day, all day, if you become extremely intolerant your pancreas can become locked in this scenario, and it will over produce insulin leaving you with slight hypoglycaemia (low blood sugar) and therefore your blood sugar levels could be permanently lower than the norm, this will make you feel sluggish and tired with little energy.

This is the pre diabetic state that extreme food intolerants often develop.

Conversely, if you do not produce enough insulin, then you will have hyperglycaemia, (high blood sugar levels) where there is a lack of insulin production by the pancreas, if you are still producing small amounts of insulin, then it may be controlled by diet and medication in tablet form, you would then be classed as a type 2 diabetic, but if your pancreas looses the ability to produce insulin altogether, then you will have to inject insulin to regulate your blood sugar levels, and will be deemed a type 1 diabetic.

Diabetes is a very complex issue and there are other factors coming into play when it comes to the causes of diabetes.

If you are full of gallstones or have a clogged liver, then many of your organs within the ribcage will be slightly enlarged, because they have not had the correct nutrients to rebuild their tissue correctly for maybe many years, they will not be functioning properly either, anyway lets assume that they have all enlarged slightly, they are and will have to compete for space within the ribcage, after all there is only so much room in there, this puts pressure on many organs, one of the areas effected will be the common bile duct, especially if you are full of gallstone,

This can become restricted, the pancreatic juices flow down and through the common bile duct, any restriction in the bile duct whatsoever, will reduce the ability of your pancreas to freely release the enzymes and hormones, if there is sufficient restriction in the common bile duct it can cause these enzymes and hormones to well up continually every day in the pancreas,

Food intolerants often feel some discomfort in their stomach after eating sugary food, this is not just the yeast overgrowth being fed, but can also be the enzymes welling up in the common bile duct and causing discomfort and even pain from the pancreas, these enzymes and hormones are extremely concentrated, and if sufficient restriction is there for long enough this will cause some of the tissue that produces these enzyme elements to be destroyed or literally dissolved, your pancreas will literally be damaged by it's own enzymes and hormones.

If the tissue that is responsible for producing insulin is destroyed (the eyelets of langerhans) then you will become diabetic.

So the possible causes of diabetes are very complex, and begins with your diet upsetting your digestive tract, too much imbalanced protein, pasteurised dairy products and sugar in your diet, causing your liver to clog, and in turn impinging on your pancreas, causing it to work very hard but very inefficiently, eventually the tissue in you pancreas which produces insulin, is degraded to the point where it cannot produce enough insulin, or non at all, you are then deemed to have a diabetic condition, either type 1 or type 2 diabetic.

Type 1 diabetics regulate their blood sugar levels with insulin injections, but type 2 diabetics produce a small amount of insulin from their pancreas, and can control insulin level by taking medication in tablet form, often the drugs prescribed will be, metformin or glyclicide

Initially your bad diet upsets the H.D.L, L.D.L and V.L.D.L clogging the liver, the consequential loss of liver function then impinges on your pancreas, then due to the lack of elements reqd to maintain and build new cells within your pancreas, your pancreas begins to degrade, especially the cells and tissue within the pancreas itself, this in turn causes problems with enzyme and hormone production, the end result is poor bile and enzyme flow down the common bile duct, and possible damage to the islets of Langerhans that produce the hormone insulin, which regulates blood sugar levels.

It's not always this chain of events that causes diabetes to develop.

Certain viruses are believed to cause pancreatic problems.

Some illnesses can cause you to develop pancreatic problems.

Many pregnant women develop diabetes, this may be because they are already advancing into food intolerance, and pregnancy tips them over the edge into the developing scenarios previously discussed, and in relation to food intolerance they are developing, a clogged liver, expanding organs competing for space etc, as the baby develops and grows it puts more pressure on the common bile duct, and the pancreas, if this is sufficiently impeded, a lack of free flow of enzymes and hormone production can ensue, this can lead to the lack of release of the hormone insulin into the blood, leaving the pregnant woman temporarily diabetic.

Although most of these women return to normal after they have given birth because they regain the ability to produce sufficient amounts of insulin again.

If these scenarios have happened to a woman then she needs to adopt the recovery programme in this book, because there is a very strong possibility that she has actually gained food intolerance, and has gallstones or at the very least a clogged liver.

There is no coming back if you develop type one insulin dependant diabetes, you have it for the rest of your life, and a strict dietary regime, along with insulin injections to control blood sugar levels, must be followed, if other organs of the body are not going to be seriously damaged.

I monitored my blood sugar level throughout recovery; it should run between 4.5 and 6. I found in the early stages that my blood sugar level ran around 2.6 to 3. This is low and could be considered hypoglycaemic, so my pancreas was producing too much insulin and holding my blood sugar levels down. This could be considered as a pre diabetic state. This state of affairs persisted, even after I tried eating no sugar at all, to try and regulate the over production, or slow down the over production of the hormone insulin.

The wheat and dairy exemption diet did not seem to have an effect in reducing the problem, it was only after completing each gallbladder and liver flush that I noticed my blood sugar levels were beginning to rise, and this rise was noticeably connected to each time I did a gallbladder and liver flush.

I now realise that the amount of gallstones and liver dysfunction I had, was causing the liver not to function properly, and this was impinging on my pancreas, and causing an imbalance, and upsetting my insulin production.

After full recovery i now run somewhere between 4.5 and 6 this is considered to be normal.

The pancreas does not repair itself as readily as the liver, and if you damage your pancreas you are often on a one-way street with no U turn.

We in the western world are eating the wrong diet.

Again the number one priority for pancreatic well-being is diet.

THE DAIRY CONNECTION

All the scenarios discussed in this chapter, in relation to the liver, pancreas and kidneys, are all responsible for the fact that, if you are intolerant to wheat, then you will also be intolerant to dairy products for some time.

This is because you don't produce the correct bile or enzymes, and your gut flora is not able to break down and absorb dairy products properly, and certain elements of the dairy products will be over absorbed and others under absorbed, such as the casein protein and the lactose in milk.

These elements then wash through the digestive tract in a relatively raw state, and toxins build up in your digestive tract, your system cannot expel these toxins because detoxification is not functioning properly, due to a clogged up liver and kidneys, and this in turn makes you feel tired and weary.

Added to this is the connection with yeast overgrowth, the lactose (milk sugar) feeds the yeast overgrowth, this is by far the most important problem, if you as a food intolerant keep ingesting large quantities of dairy products, you will feed the bad bacteria in your digestive tract, this will seriously inhibit your ability to break down food, and will leave you feeling windy, bloated, and very tired.

There is also the possibility that the thyroid has been affected, and thus you may have problems regulating the calcium from the milk, once it is in your system.

Many of the amino acids (proteins are broken down into amino acids) are required in the regulatory process of calcium by the thyroid, we intolerants have problems breaking down proteins, and thus the thyroid could have little of the correct elements to work with, and therefore regulation of calcium could be affected. Although I have to say that this is conjecture at this stage.

After about 14 months, and once recovery is well under way, these scenarios in the digestive tract recede, and dairy products may be tolerated again, although in small amounts, because they were part of the causal factors, in the failures in your digestive tract in the first place, and can never be eaten in large quantities again.

THE WHEAT CONNECTION

By far the worst reaction you will have as a food intolerant, is if you eat wheat based products, because of the pre described inabilities within of your liver and pancreas, you will not produce adequate amounts of bile and enzymes to break down the gluten, in any wheat based products.

If you adopt the recovery diet for a month or so, you will feel much better, but if you then begin to eat wheat again you will very quickly bloat, and feel very uncomfortable, you will soon decide to re adopt the recovery plan because ingesting gluten will make you feel so ill.

Gluten, the protein found in wheat is very difficult to break down, and requires large amounts of digestive enzymes from your pancreas, and lots of bile from your liver, to create the correct environment within your digestive tract to break down the gluten.

So any wheat based products, such as pizzas, pasta, bread, etc will have a serious affect on your digestive tract, if you cannot break down the gluten, then your digestive tract will begin compensation, and either give you loose bowels or constipation (IBS), depending how food intolerant you are.

THE SUGAR CONNECTION

Any raw, refined sugar within the digestive tract will feed the bad bacteria, this will seriously impede your ability to break down food, imbalancing your gut flora and making you feel bloated, especially if you have been diagnosed with diverticulitis.

Raw refined sugar is very destructive to the digestive tract of a fit and healthy person, but to a food intolerant it can have a dramatic effect on your ability to break down food. I would even suggest that refined sugar is just as destructive to your liver as alcohol.

In general fruits are all right to eat, although you should regulate you ingestion of certain fruits whilst in recovery, especially oranges, you will find this information in the list of foods you can eat.

SUMMARY

So we have lost the ability to break down wheat products.

The lactose in dairy products are upsetting our gut flora, feeding the candida, (yeast overgrowth). Any processed sugars are also feeding candida (yeast overgrowth), further upsetting gut flora.

The scenarios relating to sugar, wheat and dairy intolerance and reactions within the digestive tract, are further discussed in far more detail in "the in depth medical explanations" starting on page 248.

ASSOCIATED PROBLEMS

Many conditions now and in later life could be attributed to a high intake of wheat, dairy, and processed sugar, this clogs the liver, culminating in intolerance, and causing one or other problems.

These conditions are as a consequence of the failures within the digestive tract as described in this chapter.
Below is a list of many common conditions, which in those of us who are susceptible, are or could be attributed to gained food intolerance due to a clogged liver.

- Acid indigestion or reflux

- Acne

- Anaemia (iron deficient)

- Anxiety

- Bloating or retention
  (The whole body goes puffy and bloated, not fat but fluid retention, Michelin man effect)

- Candida Albicans

- Celiac disease
  (Only the later life celiac disease and condition)

- Crohn's disease

- Colon cancer

- Colonitis

- Dermatitis herpetiformis

- Depression

- Diabetes (late onset)

- Diverticulitis

- Fibromyalgia

- Gallstones

- Gout

- Hypoglycaemia
  (Low blood sugar)

- Headaches

- IBS

- Kidney stones

- Lower back pain
  (Especially L5 S1)

- ME
  (Myalgic Encephalitis)

- Mild arthritic symptoms

- Osteoporosis

- Pernicious anaemeia
  (Lack of B12 absorption, crohn`s disease)

- Piles

- Pre Menstrual tension

- Sinus problems

- Thyroid problems

- Thrush in women

- Ulcerative colitis

- Ulcers (Gastric and duodenal)

- Yeast overgrowth (Candida)

The lack of vitamin and mineral absorption, and the subsequent lack of synthesisation of many elements in the liver, also gives rise to other symptoms, all be it in their milder forms.

Children in some city areas are beginning to get rickets, yes rickets in our society today, this should be completely impossible in the times we live in, after all, never in the history of mankind have we had available to us all the nutrition that we have today.

Many or all of the people developing the following conditions certainly have access to the vitamins and minerals causing their problems, so why are we seeing these conditions, the foods that are available to us in the western world, should in theory make it virtually impossible for these conditions to precipitate.

Even someone on a very poor diet, is extremely unlikely not to come across the vitamins and minerals required, to prevent these conditions from developing.

It is due to the fact that they are unable to efficiently break down, and absorb the foods they are ingesting, this gives a real insight into how our western diet is affecting our digestive tract, and impeding our ability to extract nutrients from the food we are eating.

The following are beginning to be seen in some of the population.

BERIBERI

There are definite signs of old condition unheard of in this country for many years.
Beriberi Related to a lack of vitamin B1, Thiamine, can give rise to water logging of tissue, (water retention) and/or nerve damage.

RICKETS

Rickets, related to a lack of vitamin D, (Cholecalciferol), can give rise to weak bones.

Bowing of the legs is a typical sign of rickets.

SCURVY

Scurvy is related to a lack of vitamin C, (Ascorbic acid), this lack of absorption can give rise to, bleeding gums, sores, ulcers, aching joints and muscles, tooth problems, burst capillaries.

These symptoms are only clearly apparent if you are extremely intolerant, and are related to the lack of absorption of certain vitamins and minerals, such as many of the B vitamins, and even vitamin C if you are a smoker.

Many intolerants have iron deficient anaemia when they first embark on the recovery programme, that is why I advise you to take iron in early recovery.

Pernicious anaemia, caused by a lack of B12 absorption, is usually initiated by a lack of Intrinsic factor production in the stomach, and/or an inflamed terminal ileum in your digestive tract, it is unusual for food intolerants to have pernicious anaemia, but it can occur in extreme cases.

I could go on and on about problems related to lack of absorption, but I am sure you are getting the picture by now, and realising that diet and cleaning the liver is extremely important in relation to recovery.

WHAT'S WRONG WITH WHEAT PRODUCTS?

Bread made in the earlier parts of the 19th century would be made with low gluten content flour, and would not be fortified, and the yeasts used would not be the intense types we have today, this would make a much harder loaf of bread, but it would be much easier to break down by your digestive tract, and far less difficult to digest and absorb the nutrients it contained.

After 1960 wheat for bread making was mainly imported from Canada, because wheat was in very short supply in Britain during the Second World War, and for about 10 years immediately after the war.

Until 1960 we were mainly using British wheat, which had a lower gluten content, therefore after the war it took ten years or so for high gluten content Canadian wheat to be imported in large quantities to make bread from.

Thus gluten intolerance in Britain, lags behind America and Canada by about 10 years, this explains why our health problems lag behind America and Canada by 10 years, Canadian wheat has a high gluten content, and is good for bread making, it makes a fluffier lighter loaf.

OBSERVATIONS

After all the experimenting on myself, and the reactions of other people I have found with food intolerance, I am now convinced and say this damning statement with conviction, that the causal factor of most food intolerances is wheat and/or the modern flours that man produces.

When I question anyone who says they have intolerance to a particular product, I usually find after prolonged questioning of their life history and reactions to food, that strangely I inevitably arrived back at wheat products.

I have had many people who say they cannot eat dairy products, but after careful questioning, I realise that they are not just intolerant to the dairy products, but mainly the wheat products, and if you take away the wheat and dairy products, after some time maybe 14 to 18 months, and a series of gallbladder and liver flushes, they will begin to tolerate these products again, albeit in small amounts, this is a revelation to them, because if they stayed off the dairy products they felt better, but if you take the wheat away as well, they inevitably find a vast improvement in their condition.

This is one reason why I say wheat is often many peoples first intolerance, and the main cause of their other intolerances. I don't say this lightly and have several reasons for coming to this conclusion, these are all covered at some point in this book.

After analysing myself and others I have found that for some as yet unexplainable reason, gained food intolerance can give you any number of symptoms, which are listed in the symptoms chapter on pages 18 to 21, although these symptoms are very difficult to pin down to one product.

I can find definite and recognisable cases of celiac disease (the measurable flattened villi and antibody reaction to gluten in wheat), even looking back into the 1800s, although most of these cases are recorded as child born celiac.

After I first realised I was intolerant to wheat, I asked my doctor for a blood test for celiac disease I could not believe it when it came back negative.

I had all the classic symptoms, and after experimenting on others and myself for some time, I definitely pinned down the reactions to wheat, and the definite vast improvement in my and other people's condition if it was left out of our diet.

I know this, and can say it with some certainty, after the very careful study of what myself and others ate, and the reactions as detailed in the reaction chart and daily diet records on pages 30-33.

If I look back I cannot find convincing evidence of I.B.S or chronic fatigue syndrome M.E, or other wheat intolerance related conditions until the 1970s, it seems that these conditions did not become very common until the early 1970s onwards, it's either that, or the possibility that prior to this these cases were not recorded, or maybe these people were diagnosed with some other condition or illness.

FLOUR AND BREAD, OATS AND CORN

I have looked into the production of flour, and found that modern flours since around the end of the last world war have been fortified, far more than they were before.

This made me wonder if it was not just the fact that the gluten content of modern bread is hard for the body to break down, but maybe the cocktail of added elements could somehow be affecting modern man, because before these fortifying vitamins, minerals, and agents were added to flour there were very few cases of what is now seen as chronic fatigue (M.E), IBS, or indeed wheat intolerance, or celiac disease.

So I began to wonder if this wheat intolerance was a long standing very slow degrading of the digestive tract, due in some part, to the fortifying of the wheat flour since the last war.

Most modern white bread is made from what is called 70% extraction rate flour, that is to say that the flour is in the main, only a part of the milled grain, mainly the gluten protein fraction, and not the whole grain, the main reason for this is that the gluten traps pockets of carbon dioxide in the bread making process, and makes for a nice fluffy loaf of bread, which the housewife prefers to buy.

Modern breads are also fortified, the main reason for this fortification was to make sure that the general population received a good supplement of some of the more important basic vitamins, such as the B vitamins to help prevent some pre second world war conditions such as rickets and beriberi, which were quite common in the general population at that time.

Modern white bread and brown bread are high in protein; they are fortified breads with added iron, thiamine, nicotinic acid, and purified chalk.

The flour is bleached to make it whiter and not its natural yellowy colour.

Flour improvers are used to make bread more glutinous, more elastic, and whiten the bread, thus forming a softer fluffier loaf, which again the housewife wants to buy.

Other elements are also added such as genetically modified Soya, Dextrose a digestible sugar, Calcium propionate (a mould inhibitor), Stearoyl-2-lactylate speeds up fermentation, and makes dough more machine tolerant to mixing, Ammonium Chloride a nitrogen to help yeasts build proteins.

Extra gluten is often added to poor flours, one ingredient azodicarbonamide, an oxidiser, is banned in many countries, such as Canada, Japan, Australia and New Zealand.

In Britain most breads are baked using the Chorley wood process, this involves using enzymes to accelerate dough fermentation, (the proofing process), the dough is then thoroughly mixed, further accelerating the proofing process, therefore more bread can be produced in much less time, and more efficiently.

It's not fully understood how some of these improvers work, but basically they are all helping to speed up the proofing process.

Many of these elements are not fully converted after the Chorleywood process, and it is now thought by some scientific bodies, that the gluten and Soya proteins are not broken down efficiently, into a form, which the human body can effectively break down.

This pauses the first question! If we do not fully understand how these agents work then how can we possibly know what effect they will have on your digestive tract over a number of years?

White bread also contains added ingredients such as salts, fats, sugar, milk and milk products, rice, Soya, oats, enzyme preparations, preservatives, emulsifiers and stabilisers.

The problem with this modern flour concoction, is that it makes a loaf which the body finds very difficult to break down, and after years of this barrage, your digestive system begins to slowly loose the ability to continue to cope with this intensely fortified food, especially when you combine it with eating dairy products which are also difficult to break down.

This, in those of us who are susceptible, will cause our livers to clog and gain food intolerance, and can flip your digestive tract into what I call the emergency state over a couple of years in the latter stages of advanced intolerance.

If you are very intolerant to wheat, you will find that grains such as oats will also affect you, even when you are on the recovery programme.

Another grain, corn, may have affected you slightly before you embarked on this recovery programme, but you will find that once on the recovery programme you will have no intolerance to corn at all, because it has far less phosphorus and phytic acid in it.

I will now try to explain why problems begin to develop under the next heading.

MODERN YEASTS

It is now thought that many of the modern fast acting yeasts used in modern bread making processes, do not fully break down the gliadin and gluten fractions in the dough, this leaves elements in the bread which cannot be broken down by the digestive tract, the digestive tract then has to deal with these indigestible elements, after years of eating this modern bread, the digestive tract begins to degrade, and harmful yeasts begin to take over, usually candida albicans.

In the distant past, mostly before the first world war, bread was often made using slow acting yeasts such as sourdough, this acted on the dough much more slowly, and could take one and a half days to proof the bread before baking, this would convert all the gluten and gliadin in the flour, and make a loaf of bread which the digestive tract could easily break down.

It goes without saying that this bread would be much more friendly to the digestive tract, with no long term destructive potential to intestinal processes, these loaves of bread would be much harder, but much friendlier.

ANAEMIA, IRON AND CALCIUM

Wheat, Corn and Oats all contain phosphorus, which is in a combined form called phytic acid, this in large quantities and in particular in the more intense grains such as wheat, can hinder the absorption of calcium and iron in the digestive system, I will now try to explain my theory of the reasons why.

When making bread the phytic acid combines with calcium and iron and forms insoluble salts called phytates, these phytates are present in the dough, before it is baked.

In this state or form the calcium and iron could not be extracted and absorbed by the digestive tract, the human body has not got the ability to break it down when it is in the form of dough.

However most of these phytates, about 85%, are broken down during the proofing, heating and baking process of the dough by phytases, this then releases and makes about 85% of the iron and calcium available to the body, but this still leaves some 15% of these insoluble salts or phytates, washing through your digestive tract every day, unavailable to the body in the form of locked off iron and calcium, and these have to be processed and eradicated safely by the digestive tract.

WE NOW HAVE FOUR PROBLEMS HERE.

Problem No 1
This is loading and stressing your digestive tract every day, because it is very difficult to break down the elements in the bread, but more importantly your digestive tract has to control, recognise and expel the 15% of the locked up calcium and iron which is still in the form of phytates, and cannot be broken down or extracted.

Problem No 2
Again with regard to the calcium, iron and the phytic acid connection, this could not only be a problem for the body because some of it would be washing through the digestive tract as phytates unavailable to the body, but there is the distinct possibility that this unabsorbable or locked off calcium and iron, could possibly interfere with, and cause absorption problems with the 85% of calcium and iron, which was successfully converted by the phytases, during the bread making, and baking process into a form which the digestive tract could break down and absorb.

Problem No 3
There is a strong possibility that the absorption of other vitamins and minerals, especially in the duodenum and jejunum part of the digestive tract will also be impaired if these conditions prevail, because your digestive tract is having to try and extract vitamins and minerals, whilst trying to expel the excess locked up iron and calcium in the form of phytates, these vitamins and minerals include many B vitamins, and even vitamin C, and possibly more importantly vitamin E which is an antioxidant and helps to prevent tissue from breaking down within the digestive tract.

Problem no 4
This could also explain why many intolerants are anaemic before starting the recovery programme, this would explain the anaemia in the more advanced cases of intolerance, because one of the elements we cannot extract and absorb properly is iron, so we have the phytic acid problem, plus we intolerants are not producing enough bile and hormones from the liver and pancreas, therefore we are far less likely to be able to control the environment in our digestive tract, and extract elements from the food we eat.

OTHER POSSIBLE PROBLEMS

If there is iron washing through your digestive tract all the time because some of it is locked off from the body in the form of phytic acid, it could impair or interfere with the absorption of vitamin E, because iron impairs E absorption and E impairs iron absorption, E is extremely important in detoxification and an antioxidant, vitamin E is vital for the prevention of breakdown of tissue throughout the body.

I was patently not utilising vitamin E properly. Vitamin E was the one element that had a dramatic effect on recovery and the reaction to it even when taken in very small amounts (400iu) once every three weeks in early stages, made my eyesight more acute, my hearing more acute, and my sense of well being and awareness was improved within hours.

As I said before Vitamin E is an important antioxidant and vital for the prevention of breakdown of tissue, and it is also required in aiding the detoxification processes in the body. Some of the calcium would also be unavailable, because of the high protein content of the bread. High protein levels leech calcium from the bones, this would explain the apparent lack of calcium absorption in the advanced stages of the condition, and added to this the magnesium levels required to keep this large amount of calcium in suspension in your blood would only be there in small quantities.

Another important vitamin is Vitamin D, there also appears to be problems with the absorption of vitamin D, there are even cases of young people with mild signs of rickets in our modern society.

With all the varied foods we eat, it should be virtually impossible for anyone in 2012 to suffer from rickets; again this is probably due to poor absorption within the digestive tract.

Your thyroid gland requires calcium to work with, so there is the distinct possibility that these scenarios could also affect thyroid function.

Again considering the fortification aspect of the 70% extraction flour, as discussed earlier, with regard to the high gluten protein, some people (Celiacs) have a definite and measurable reaction to the gluten protein fraction of the wheat grain, and present with clinical symptoms, they have flattened villi in their digestive tract, and produce antibodies against the gluten, which can be detected with a blood test.

This very hard to break down gluten protein content of bread obviously causes a problem for celiacs, but it also causes problems for those of us who are not celiac, we do not have these measurable reactions, but we do share many of the celiac symptoms, many of which are listed in the symptoms chapter on pages 18 to 21.

Other more serious digestive tract problems such as ulcerative colitis, colon cancer, Crohn's disease, diverticulitis, gout etc could also be as a consequence of the wheat related scenarios in this chapter.

So if this state of affairs exists with regard to wheat, it may go some way to explaining why there seems to be a very slow degrading of the digestive tract and related organs, culminating in the digestive tract loosing its ability to process and break down foods, and causing possible bowel disorders, and the reactive states which will be described further on in this book, as covered in the "what happens to the digestive tract" chapter

ALTERNATIVES TO MODERN WHEAT

There are alternatives to using the modern wheat varieties.

- Spelt

- Kamut, relative of Durum wheat

- Einkorn

- Emmer

- Buckwheat

Spelt may be used to make home baked bread, has a similar protein fraction but does not appear to effect food intolerants, unless they have become extremely wheat intolerant.

Kamut a relative of durum wheat does not appear to react with wheat intolerants or celiacs.

Einkorn and Emmer are very old wheat varieties, and although they contain gliadin and gluten they do not appear to react with wheat intolerants, especially if left to proof for one and a half days, it is also advisable to make bread from these flours using sourdough.

EXPERIMENT

To give you an indication of the glutinous elasticity properties of bread, try taking the crust off a slice of bread, and then kneading the rest of the slice with a few drops of water.

You would think that bread would readily absorb water, but it doesn't, especially after kneading it, see how elastic and stretchy it becomes, its like putty, this is mainly due to the gluten (protein) content of the bread.

This is extremely difficult for your digestive tract to break down; your body needs to be running at 100% efficiency, to effectively deal with this modern form of bread.

This experiment will probably put you off eating bread, especially when you see the bread in this state.

CONCLUSION

So as you can see modern bread is far removed from the unleavened bread that was made in the not so distant past. Unleavened bread is basically made from just mixing rough milled flour, using all of the grain, with water or beer, and then baking it. This bread is hard and unattractive, and not nice to the pallet, you have just baked a brick.

But and this is a big but, a lot of the protein, iron, calcium, and other recently added elements would not be there in large amounts, and therefore the digestive tract would find this a lot easier to break down and digest, therefore it goes without saying that this bread would be much friendlier to the digestive tract, although there would not be as much potential protein energy value in it, or anywhere near as much theoretic energy in it persae, but you would probably extract more energy from the unleavened bread than our modern breads, because we would be able to fully break down and utilise these un bastardised breads, at least you would be extracting and absorbing a natural and balanced amount of these nutrients.

Unless your digestive tract is working at full capacity, it will not be able to break down these intensive modern breads and pastas, even a fully functioning digestive tract will have difficulty expelling the unwanted fractions and toxins produced by these modern breads, and at the same time manage to extract some energy from this concoction of elements.

Many of the aspects covered in this chapter can only be assumptions, as this is a very complex issue, and to unravel the exact molecular or biological interactions that cause complications in the digestive tract could take a lifetime, or indeed never be fully understood.

As I've said before, the main problem with wheat, is that it is processed and fortified and in most of the products we eat, and after some years of this barrage, our digestive tract and other organs degrade and clog up, loosing the ability to break down and absorb many foods, mainly wheat and dairy products.

I would not advise you to buy gluten free bread, most of these alternatives contain yeasts, large amounts of carbohydrate, and other additives, which will affect your digestive tract, I have experimented with many of these gluten free breads, and found that they affect intolerants. I tried these alternative breads on quite a few intolerants I was treating, and found that all of them reacted to one degree or another, usually it gave them stomach ache and bloating, these symptoms persisted until they had cleaned there liver and kidneys.

This is a quite a radical statement, but I would go as far as to say that; high wheat based products such as pizza, pasta, and in particular bread, should carry a health warning stating that over indulgence, over a lengthy period of time, can lead to health problems in later life.

Babies should not be weaned onto high protein wheat based products until they are at least 16 to 18 months old, their digestive tract will not have developed sufficiently to break down the high gluten protein content of these products, even after this they should only be fed small amounts of wheat based products and not every day.

If we all ate wheat-based products in small amounts, in unprocessed form, and not every day the wheat would not pause or cause a problem.

ACKNOWLEDGMENT

After feeling tired + bloated for many years. I had a conversation with Mr Wrathall who questioned me about my health over my lifetime. He then advised me to adopt his advised diet which included the gallbladder flush. After one month I noticed a vast improvement in energy and felt far less tired. I would advise anyone to read his book because it has certainly helped me recover. A new lease of life.

Mr G Bloundlale

WHAT'S WRONG WITH DAIRY PRODUCTS?

After months of staying off wheat, I found that I had to stay off dairy products as well, as this also had a reaction, and I could not recover digestive function and control yeast overgrowth, until wheat and dairy products and also refined sugar were eliminated.

PROBLEMS WITH DAIRY PRODUCTS

As I see it there are five main problems with dairy products.

1 Almost all of the good bacteria and enzymes have been killed off in the pasteurising process.

2 Much of calcium in milk is not being absorbed.

3 Milk contains lactose (milk sugar).

4 Dairy products are in too many foods.

5 They are mucous building

Lets look at these aspects in a little more detail.

1 Almost all of the good bacteria and enzymes have been killed off, along with the bad bacteria, during the pasteurising process.

This leaves the digestive tract with all the work to do, as there is very little help from the natural bacteria and enzymes, the digestive tract has to produce more bile and enzymes to break it down, this is stressful to the digestive tract.

This is a catch 22 Scenario, because we want to eradicate some of the bad bacteria from milk such as Brucellos (Genus Brucella) and Tuberculosis by it, but we are unwittingly making the milk much more difficult to break down, dramatically increasing the workload of the digestive tract, if your digestive tract is compromised even slightly then you will not be able to break down dairy products efficiently.

2 There is a quite a lot of calcium in dairy products, but we don't appear to be absorbing it properly, there is also quite a lot of calcium added to our modern breads, this means there is possibly an excess of calcium in our digestive tract, this would require large amounts of magnesium in our diets to keep the calcium in suspension, and because of poor absorption there may not be enough Vit D to aid in absorbing the calcium, and there will definitely not be enough magnesium in our modern diet to keep this amount of calcium in suspension, this could lead to calciate type kidney stones.

The lack of breakdown and absorption of calcium means parathyroid function could also be affected, as calcium is one element the parathyroid gland requires for the regulation of many systems in your body.

There is also the possibility that osteoporosis could develop in later life, because you will loose some of the ability to extract, absorb, suspend and process the calcium within your digestive tract.

Lets put it this way, why, if there is so much calcium in the modern diet, are there so many people with osteoporosis, thyroid problems, kidney stones etc, surely there should be little sign of these conditions, patently we are not breaking down extracting or absorbing, or utilizing this calcium efficiently.

Many dieticians absolutely tear my recovery diet to pieces, saying there is not enough calcium in the diet, this is a complete fallacy, there is more than enough calcium in the advised diet, and more importantly your digestive tract will be working more efficiently, and more able to extract and utilise this calcium.

Virtually all the animals on the planet only drink milk in infancy, so how do you think they maintain bones throughout the rest of their lives, yes exactly, they extract it from the foods they eat, there is enough calcium in other sources of food without them drinking milk, alternative sources of calcium are found in all leafy green vegetables, fish and eggs.

3 An extremely important factor relating to dairy products in the case of gained intolerance, is the lactose (milk sugars).

Almost invariably people with intolerance have yeast overgrowth, and the lactose (milk sugar) feeds the yeast overgrowth, (candida).

This is the main reason for taking dairy products out of the diet in the case of food intolerance.

I usually find that people can cope with plain live or bio yoghurt, because the bacteria used to make live yoghurt have converted the lactose into lactic acid, and to some degree separated the dairy protein casein, and it was the lactose (milk sugar) and to a lesser degree the casein protein causing a problem, and not the other elements in the milk.

Plain live or Bio yoghurt contains lactobacillus bulgaricus, biofidous, and streptococcus lactis, these are helpful in regaining good gut flora, and therefore it is recommended to take live or Bio yoghurt every day, in the unlikely event it reacts with you once you are on the recovery programme, just take it out of your diet again and take a pro biotic supplement instead, do not take live yoghurt and pro biotics together or you may get constipation.

4 They are in many foods, and eaten in many cases at every meal in one form or another, this again puts stress on the digestive tract.

Just look at the labels on the products you buy every day, and you will be amazed at how many dairy products you are ingesting every day, and in many cases ingesting them at every meal.

5 Dairy products also cause an excess amounts of mucus to build up in your system, clogging up certain organs and impairing their function.

Sinus problems are often related to dairy intake, this is due to the excess mucous forming in the sinus tubes.

Many singers do not eat dairy products, because they have learned through experience that they are mucus forming, and can impair their vocal ability, and lung capacity.

DAIRY AND GLUTEN CONNECTION

Even as a baby we are fed dairy products, often powdered milk, which is hard for a baby to break down, little wonder that many babies throw back most of the milk fed to them in powdered form, as apposed to breast fed babies, who in general find no problem digesting breast milk.

It is known that Celiacs (people with a measurable intolerance to gluten in wheat) often cannot cope with dairy products for very complicated reasons, of which we need not look into here, although this intolerance in celiacs often goes away after 12 to 14 months of recovery.

Those of us who are intolerant to wheat, but are not celiac have the same scenario, in that we too cannot cope with dairy products until about 12 to 14 months into recovery. We both have the same intolerance, but the Celiac scenario is measurable in that they have antibody reaction and flattened villi and we do not.

There are some theories surrounding the intolerance to dairy products In celiacs, one such theory which may hold some truth, is the fact that in modern farming methods, dairy cows are fed gluten containing cereal grains, and the theory goes that the gluten is imparted into the milk, and we make many of our dairy based cheeses, yoghurts, cakes etc from this milk, and therefore a celiac may be inadvertently ingesting wheat, or to be more precise, gluten. Although I have to say that this view, and theoretic connection, in my view, is a little tenuous to say the least.

The previous factors as discussed earlier in this chapter in relation to dairy products, are the major reasons why you have an inability to digest, or cope with dairy products in the early stages of recovery.

The other major reason why you loose the ability to cope with dairy products is the fact that you have gained food intolerance, through your over ingestion of wheat, sugar, and dairy products over a lifetime, this has clogged your liver and possibly given you gallstones, the consequential lack of bile enzyme and hormone production leaves you less able to break down dairy products, thus your digestive tract will to some degree treat dairy products as toxic, and try to evacuate them from your digestive tract.

REACTIONS

Be very careful with dairy products if you are very intolerant and in the early stages of recovery, if you stepped off the recovery programme and treated yourself to an ice cream on lets say Sunday afternoon, it will make you tired until about Thursday afternoon, a cup of milk will do the same, any dairy product will have the same reaction in the first 12 to 14 months of recovery. This is partly due to the toxins produced, also you are feeding your yeast overgrowth, which will thrive off the lactose in the milk, and cause an upset in your gut flora.

The only exception to this is live or Bio yoghurt, make sure its plain live or Bio yoghurt, and not strawberry or flavoured and possibly sweetened live or Bio yoghurt, and only eat an average serving every day, don't go mad with it just because its something you can eat.

I felt I had to say this because I have found people having two 500g tubs of live yoghurt a day, this is total over indulgence, and will give you digestive reaction.

If you are very intolerant in the early stages of recovery, you may have a very porous digestive tract, and you may not even be able to cope with the live yoghurt. So try some in the early stages of recovery and judge the reaction for yourself.

If the small amount I recommended taking reacts with you, then take it out of your diet, take pre and pro biotics instead, as prescribed by your health shop.

Your ability to detoxify is limited when you are in the depths of intolerance. The dairy products can cause toxins and mucous to build up, and your immune system, lymph, liver, and kidneys, can't eradicate them fast enough, this will trip you into toxic overload and, make you feel tired, its nature trying to buy some time by putting you to sleep yet again, so it can do some repairs, and obviously whilst your asleep you won't be eating anything to further add to the toxic load on your system.

CONCLUSION

So, in the case of dairy products we are eating far too many of them every day.

This is adding to the load on the digestive tract, clogging up many systems in our bodies, causing toxins and mucous to build, and helping to create the failures in the digestive tract, it is not solely the causal factor of food intolerance for many people, it is part of the food intolerance phenomena.

The failures in the digestive tract, as described in "the in depth medical explanations" starting on page 248, are responsible for the inability to digest dairy products, in the first 12 months, to 2 years months of recovery.

Once fully recovered dairy products may be tolerated, but don't eat too many of them, eat small amounts and definitely not every day.

Everything in moderation as many of my clients keeps telling me.

ACKNOWLEDGMENT

I decided to try the diet after suffering years of discomfort and tiredness. I had almost given up any hope of feeling better. My problems went back to when I was at school, but it wasn't until I started to get better that I realised how ill I had been.

My energy didn't come back overnight though, but after 18 months on the diet I feel about 75% back to where I should be.

The greatest improvement came after about 4 gallstone flushes, and I intend to keep up with the flushes until the stones stop coming. Yeast overgrowth has been the most difficult part to control. The yeast thrives on all the foods I enjoy. Cutting out chocolate, mushrooms, beer and wine is not my idea of fun, but slowly over several months I did get on top of the problem. It seemed necessary to get rid of the gallstones first to be able to control the yeast. Now that the stomach pains have gone it is clearly noticeable if I eat any foods with wheat or sugar in them.

My experiences have taught me how important it is to eat a balanced diet. I think years of eating large amounts of bread and very little veg made things worse for me.

I do find it worrying that most G.P.'s know very little about dietary problems. My doctor told me that I had I.B.S. and that I would have to put up with it, just like about 20% of the population. I had a scan for gallstones and was told that I definitely had not got any. Since then I have flushed about 200 stones out!

I would recommend trying the diet and flushes to anyone suffering similar symptoms because it has made such a difference to me. If you don't feel well for whatever reason then there must be something causing it and chances are that you can do something about it. I am certain that many illnesses are either caused or exaggerated by diet, and I feel that the medical profession has a great deal to learn yet.

WHAT'S WRONG WITH CARBOHYDRATE?

Processed or raw sugar is a major problem in the modern diet; it is in virtually everything we eat.

Next time you come home after shopping, take aside all the products that contain processed or raw sugar, you will be amazed at the amount of foods that have sugar in them, it will probably surprise you to find just how much processed sugar you are inadvertently ingesting every day, usually at every meal. This should set alarm bells ringing, so we will just have a quick look at some of the problems this sugar can pause within the body and digestive tract.

DIGESTIVE PROBLEMS AND SUGAR

If you eat processed carbohydrate (sugar), your digestive tract will very quickly absorb it, you can not possibly burn this sugar at the rate it is able to be absorbed by your digestive system, so you will automatically store some of this as glycogen in your liver, or convert it into fat.
This is the major problem with processed sugar, it gives you a short burst of energy because you absorb it very quickly, the rest is put into storage, and then you will be left feeling weary and weak.

Carbohydrate can be found in many natural foods, mainly fruit, most vegetables also contain carbohydrate such as carrots and potatoes, this is friendly carbohydrate, and if you are fit and healthy this type of carbohydrate does not pose a problem, but if you have gained food intolerance you will probably have yeast overgrowth, in which case you will have to avoid, or eat small amounts of the very sugary fruits, as listed in the "foods you can" eat chapter, why? because these high carbohydrate containing foods will feed your yeast overgrowth or candida. Therefore it is very important to stay away from the fruits I advise you not to eat, until well into recovery, usually until some gallbladder and liver flushes have been completed.

So why is carbohydrate found in fruit and vegetables all right, and processed carbohydrate so destructive.

If you ingest processed carbohydrate (sugar) you are giving your system the sugar, it does not have to extract it from a food source, therefore it is very quickly absorbed and in a slightly different form than the sugars found in natural foods, in effect you are giving your body the sugar, without your digestive tract having to work for it, so in recovery any processed foods are automatically excluded, because you can virtually guarantee that if it is processed, it will contain sugar, (raw carbohydrate).

But if we now look at natural foods that contain carbohydrate, such as fruit and vegetables, your body has to break down these foods and extract the sugars from the food, these foods also contain fibre, which helps to regulate the uptake of the carbohydrate, this is a completely different concept to eating processed carbohydrate, (sugar) and is far more beneficial to your body, and far more natural, you are not giving it to your body, your digestive tract has to work to extract it, this is an essential and important difference which you need to remember whenever you eat.

If you have clogged your liver, and lost some of your ability to produce and freely pass bile, another problem develops relating to the absorption of carbohydrate, you will not be able to break down oils fats and proteins efficiently, and therefore your body will effectively turn to the carbohydrate for sustenance, so in the main it will be forced to live off this processed carbohydrate, therefore we need to control this situation if recovery is to take place. This is another reason why it is so important to follow the recovery diet; we need to keep a balance in your digestive system between oils and fats, proteins and carbohydrates whilst in recovery.

You require some natural carbohydrate, from fruit and vegetables, to help maintain a healthy gut flora, and break down and digest other foods that do not contain sugars, such as the oils fats and proteins, but it is very important to ingest these carbohydrates as the diet suggests, to maintain a balanced gut flora whilst in recovery.

The speed at which sugars are absorbed in the digestive tract is measured by a system called the "glycaemic index" this basically is a measure of the speed at which any given sugar in food, or sugar itself is absorbed into your system.

For instance processed sugar or honey have a very high glycaemic index, about as high as you can get, but natural foods such as fruit and vegetables usually release their sugars far more slowly.

Its often said that you should stay away from high glycaemic index foods, but this is not necessarily the case, many high glycaemic index foods are generally all right as long as they are in their natural state as fruit or vegetables, The exception to this rule is oranges, do not eat oranges until recovery is well under way, you should always stay away from are the high glycaemic processed carbohydrates (raw sugars), as in chocholate, toffee, jelly etc.

Sugar in the modern diet is very destructive and disruptive to the correct functioning of the digestive tract.

If you ingest too much processed carbohydrate (sugar), your entire digestive tract will slightly change the way it functions, it will absorb readily the sugar but this excess of sugar imbalances your digestive system, your digestive tract will literally be awash with sugar, this will inevitably therefore interfere with your natural gut flora, thus consequently there will be an imbalance in the good and bad bacteria and, therefore efficient digestion cannot take place, you will not create the correct environment in your digestive tract to break down difficult foods such as oils, fats, and proteins efficiently, even if your liver is working correctly and not clogged, and you have a free flow of bile enzymes and hormones down your common bile duct, you will still have imbalanced gut flora.

Other issues relate to the over ingestion of processed sugar, the previously mentioned upset gut flora leads to malabsorption of vitamins, minerals, and trace elements.

One of the major problems of over ingestion of sugar when linked with the over ingestion of dairy products and gluten protein, is the effect it has on the cholesterol molecules H.D.L, L.D.L, and V in your blood, in that it will distort the balance of these molecules and cause you to gain raised cholesterol production by the liver, the processes involved in this reaction can be better understood if you read chapter 13, page 120.

THE LIVER AND SUGAR

In a healthy person insulin is produced by the pancreas, and stimulates the uptake of glucose into the liver and muscle cells.

When your liver is clogged and compromised it has little storage capacity for sugar (glycogen), you may be producing insulin, but the reduced capacity for storage in the liver means that blood sugars have nowhere to be stored other than conversion to fat or to a large degree utilised by muscles, and therefore the pancreas has to produce large amounts of insulin every day, all day, in a constant attempt to store the excess sugar ingested from our modern diet.

Exercise and daily activity burns off some of this excess glucose, but when blood sugars dip, there may be little backup in the liver of stored sugar (glycogen) if your liver is clogged, then blood sugar levels cannot be maintained, and dip slightly, causing you to feel weak and tired.

CARBOHYDRATE AND DIABETES

Another and crucial issue in relation to, yes I'm going to say it again, processed carbohydrate (raw sugar), is the fact that your blood will very quickly become filled with glucose, this may give you a burst of energy, but there is one organ of the body that will have to go into overdrive every day, especially with our modern diet, and that is the pancreas.

One of the hormones your pancreas produces is insulin, which your body utilises to regulate the glucose levels in your blood. If you ingest too much sugar at every meal, as most people in the western world un-knowingly do, you can obviously see that your pancreas will have to work like a lunatic to keep up with the production of insulin, to regulate blood glucose levels.

If this situation is sustained for a number of years, the pancreas can become programmed over time, to produce large amounts of insulin constantly, and if food or sugar is not ingested for three or four hours, then the over production of insulin can induce a dip in blood sugar levels, you then become slightly low in blood sugars (hypoglycaemic). This may leave you feeling weak, tired and shaky. This situation is often deemed to indicate a pre-diabetic state, in that blood sugar levels often run low at regular intervals throughout the day.

You can then begin over time, and as the Pancreas degrades, to move into a constantly high (hyperglycaemic) state, constantly high blood sugar levels, this is because your pancreas can become exhausted over a number of years, and does not produce enough insulin to keep up with the intake of carbohydrate, You would then be deemed to be diabetic, and require medication with insulin to regulate your blood sugar levels.

This is partly, notice I say partly the cause of diabetes; it is definitely not the sugar alone causing the problem.

Diabetes is a condition where the islets of langerhans in the pancreas have lost the ability to produce enough or any insulin at all, to regulate and keep blood sugar levels within certain parameters.

Diabetes is literally beginning to acquire epidemic proportions in the western world.

You can read more about the causes of diabetes in chapter 13 page 125.

If you become a type 1 Diabetic, your pancreas has lost the ability to produce any insulin at all, so the regulatory hormone insulin, for blood glucose regulation, has gone, therefore you will have to inject insulin every day, and be very careful with your diet to keep blood glucose levels stable.

Diabetics have to test their blood glucose levels at particular points during the day and then decide how much insulin they may require to keep their blood sugar levels stable.

This system works on a scale, low or no glucose in the blood =0 and the more blood glucose you have in your blood the higher will be the reading.

Normal blood glucose levels are between 4.5 and 6.5 mmol/L.

If a Diabetics sugar level drops below one then he will loose coordination and even collapse, if he is not given some glucose to raise his or her blood sugar level they may descend into a coma and in the extreme even die.

If his or her blood glucose levels are consistently high, he or she will feel tired and unwell, some of the first signs and symptoms of the onset of the diabetic condition are, a severe thirst and a constant desire to urinate.

This is often the case before a diabetic is diagnosed as diabetic, if your blood sugar level is too high for a lengthy period of time, many organs of the body will definitely be damaged, circulatory, and eye problems are the usual complications, blindness and limb amputation can be the worst case scenarios.

As I said before it isn't just an excess sugar intake that is causing many people to develop diabetes, it's a combination of factors involving our modern diet and the effect this has on other organs of the body, mainly the liver, this is further explained in the chapter, "what happens to the digestive tract" page 100.

HISTORY AND CARBOHYDRATE

It is not natural to eat raw sugar, when we were wandering around in our natural environment for maybe 2,000,000 yrs, we did not eat raw sugar, we were nomads eating fruits, berries, and vegetables grubbed up from the ground, this natural carbohydrate would be the only carbohydrate we would ingest.

About the only exception to this rule would be if we stumbled across a Bees nest, and ate the honey from it.

We have only ingested processed carbohydrate in vast quantities for the last 50 to 120 yrs, if you think your digestive tract can cope with this change in diet over one or two generations, then you are deluding yourself.

There is no way our digestive tract can adapt in such little time, to this vast change in our diet. It takes hundreds of generations to adapt, definitely not 2 or 3.

CONCLUSION

Well I hope this has scared you a little and given you enough reason to stay away from processed sugar, you have to realise the importance of the potentially destructive nature of PROCESSED SUGAR.

I would even go so far as to say, "refined sugar is as destructive as alcohol".

HELICOBACTER PYLORI

- The symptoms of Helicobacter Pylori are;

- Stomach cramping.

- General stomach ache.

- Gnawing feeling in stomach area.

- Acid reflux

There is a possibility you could have Helicobacter Pylori, and this will have to be eradicated, in those of us with food intolerance to help us recover.

Up to 40% of the population may have helicobacter pylori, but it does not pause a problem if your digestive tract is healthy, it only begins to cause problems if there is digestive dysfunction.

This bacterium in those of us with food intolerance will cause stomach-ache, cramping in your stomach, and possibly stomach or duodenal ulcers.

The usual treatment is to kill off this stomach bacterium with antibiotics; this is not good, because people with food intolerance already have poor gut flora in their digestive tract as it is, and the use of these antibiotics further upsets our balance of bacteria, and gut flora, and can make any yeast overgrowth (candida) even worse.

If the symptoms are present it is important to test for this very early on in the recovery programme, there is no alternative to the use of antibiotics, because we need to eradicate the Helicobacter Pylori before recovery can take place, we will just have to accept the consequential upset in gut flora as a slight setback in the early stages of recovery.

You can't control it with diet once it has taken over, so we have to eradicate it, and a simple blood test at your doctors can identify the bacteria, and a course of antibiotics will eliminate it, then we can get on and begin to repair your digestive tract again.

WARNING

If you find you have Helicobacter Pylori, and are treated for it, the pains and aches may go away, but do not be tempted to think that you have found the answer to your stomach problems and eliminated them.

The Helicobacter Pylori has only multiplied and taken off in the first place, as a direct consequence of the upset in your gut flora, due to gained food intolerance, and the consequential inability to break down food.

If you think your cured, you are not, and months, or even years later, you will begin to fall back again into the mire of your food intolerances, and an upset stomach and bowels.

YEAST OVERGROWTH OR CANDIDA ALBICANS

WHAT IS YEAST OVERGROWTH / CANDIDA ALBICANS?

In this text I will refer to Candida Albicans as yeast overgrowth, this covers a wide range of related fungal and yeast infections under one umbrella, without the need to complicate matters by looking at specific infection types.

- Symptoms

- Whitish yellow tongue

- Bloating of the stomach

- Athletes foot

- Vaginal thrush

- Penile matter

- Also as will be explained further in the book, I include, Athletes foot and thick toenails as yeast overgrowth, also fungal infections.

The best measure of whether you have yeast overgrowth is to look at your tongue and if it is covered in a whitish, yellowish, furry, mould type substance there is a strong possibility you have developed yeast overgrowth.

Almost all food intolerants, up to 98% have yeast overgrowth.

Often there are other conditions that may proliferate, which are also an indication of yeast overgrowth, and an upset in your gut flora, such as thick toenails, Athletes foot, fungal infections, and even Thrush in women, or a creamy yellowish discharge of matter under the foreskin of the penis in males.

Yeast overgrowth is such a common condition that it could be nature's way of changing the digestive tract slightly when it is in crisis, to help it to cope with ingested imbalanced, unnatural processed foods.

Although I cannot unravel the complex possibilities, it could be that this is some kind of emergency state that the body adopts, because it is so common in people who have wheat, dairy and general food intolerance.

It is not wholly recognised as a medically definable measurable condition, because it is not too far removed from what is considered to be normal gut flora, and therefore has no diagnosable datum point.

So yeast overgrowth is not a disease or condition in its own right, but a side effect of digestive problems, either medical or food intolerance related.

This imbalance of bacteria and yeasts, will interfere and compete with normal gut flora and therefore affect digestion of food, and will to some degree thrive, multiply and live on some of the foods you eat, especially sugar, and therefore you will obtain little benefit or energy from these foods, these foods include Wine, Mouldy Cheese, Mushrooms, sugar etc, the foods that will feed the yeast overgrowth are listed at the end of this chapter.

INTESTINAL MICROBES AND HEALTH

There are billions of micro organisms in your digestive tract, these are minute life forms of differing kinds, if you have yeast overgrowth the consequential upset in gut flora will inhibit the ability of these microbes to proliferate.

They are absolutely essential for the correct breakdown of food within your intestine, they also play a pivotal roll in overall bodily function and health, it is now known that an imbalance in these intestinal microbes can cause effects in the entire body, which you would not expect.

It can affect your mood and emotion, your feeling of well being, your libido, strength, and ability to think clearly, autistic children are known to have fewer intestinal microbes, and improve measurably, if the environment in their digestive tract is also improved.

Physical and skeletal problems such as osteo and rheumatoid arthritis, joint pain, muscle cramps, lower back pain, and general stiffness, can also be improved if microbial activity in the bowel is increased, dietary changes are the main influence on these microbes, and if the dietary advice in this book is followed, a marked change in many of these symptoms and conditions is very quickly observed.

This is due to the bowel recovering a more normal gut flora, and regaining the correct PH, which is vital for the correct function of enzymes, enabling food to be broken down more efficiently and effectively, Vital B vitamins then become more available due to the recovery of the duodenum (the first part of your digestive tract).

WHAT CAUSES YEAST OVERGROWTH

There is always a causal factor with this condition, you don't catch, acquire, or develop yeast overgrowth or Candida for no reason, outside factors affecting, or influencing gut flora are responsible.

Normally the intestine is populated with millions of good and bad bacteria, this environment is normal, with normally occurring gut bacteria.

There are many types of bad bacteria, but in a normal intestinal environment this bacteria is kept in check, and causes no threat to your digestive tract, nevertheless some of this bad bacteria is necessary and required in your digestive tract, to control invasion by alien parasites, and to help in breaking down food in the digestive tract.

Good or friendly bacteria are required for the breakdown of foods, along with bile and enzymes from the liver and pancreas.

If the digestive tract is constantly upset by intolerance to certain foods, or the taking of antibiotics on numerous occasions, the normal balance of the intestine can be upset.

Every time you visit your doctor and are prescribed antibiotics it upsets the balance of bacteria and in your digestive tract, killing off some good bacteria along with the bad, especially if broadband antibiotics are used.

In someone whose immune system is already under pressure from bad diet, gained intolerance to certain foods, or an illness, this can be catastrophic, and can allow the bad bacteria to begin to colonise your digestive tract in larger amounts than would be considered normal, and become more dominant, not enough good bacteria are able to thrive to keep the bad bacteria in check.

If these conditions persist then the bad bacteria can over colonise your digestive tract, and can begin to compromise normal digestive function.

Once this bacterium has become dominant, it can be very difficult to re stabilise normal gut flora. But in the instances I have come across I am quite sure that in the first instance the overwhelming causal factor and threat to the tract has been an intolerance to some foods, or more to the point an over indulgence of many of the intolerance foods over a lifetime. Normally the first being wheat, the second dairy products, and the third processed sugar, this in turn can cause secondary intolerance to other foods such as oranges, melon etc as listed under other intolerance foods on page 45, or the cut out wall chart on page 14.

By far the greatest reason why people gain yeast overgrowth, is the fact that they have clogged their liver, the consequent lack of vitamin and mineral absorption and interaction leaves us less able to produce and maintain good gut flora.

The vast majority of people with imbalanced gut flora, have yeast overgrowth because they cannot maintain the balance of good and bad bacteria in their digestive tract, due to incorrect PH (acidity) in their digestive tract, caused by a lack of bile and enzyme production from the liver and pancreas.

TREATMENT IN RELATION TO DIET

If you want to control bacterial and or yeast overgrowth, it is no good to try and eradicate it on its own, because something has caused the conditions to exist to allow it taking over in the first place.

So we have to look at the past and your past history, and can usually unearth an intolerance to some foods, which you may not even realise you have. Strangely I find that in most cases it's usually wheat, and other foods listed on pages 42-45 or refer to the cut out wall chart on page 14.

The treatment for this condition is going to have to be done along with additional measures, other than just staying off wheat, dairy products, and processed sugars, you will have to recover your liver and kidneys, as detailed in the liver flush and kidney cleanse chapters. Only then will you be able to regain a correct gut flora.

There is a list of additional foods to be avoided at the end of this chapter, and some suggestions of what to eat, to aid in killing off the yeast overgrowth.

Symptoms will begin to dissipate once you begin to eat the right foods, but it will not die away and stay away just because you eat the right diet, or treat it with the traditional, garlic, onions, propolis, vitamin C, etc.

I have found that if you take away the intolerance foods, and keep off the toxins your digestive function slowly begins to return to normal, and the yeast overgrowth slowly dies away, even if small quantities of natural sugars as in pineapple, grapefruit, pears, bananas, apples and many other fruits are ingested.

Pineapple and grapefruit contain enzymes beneficial to the digestive tract although they may cause a reaction in early recovery if eaten in large quantities, so if you are extremely food intolerant, then small amounts should be eaten.

Apples, pears and bananas are tolerated once recovery is under way, that is why these products are not included under the # symbol on the "foods that can be eaten" list on pages 48-49, and the cut out wall chart on page 15, any of the other foods carrying this symbol # may be eaten after 2 months on the recovery diet, but only in small quantities, otherwise they will feed the yeast overgrowth.

TAKE NOTE, don't eat the fruits that you are allowed to eat in large quantities, like they are going out of fashion, or they will definitely feed the yeast overgrowth.

It's important to realise that if you keep ingesting the foods you are intolerant to, i.e. the wheat and dairy products, you will find it very difficult to control the yeast overgrowth, it will die back slightly if you take garlic, onions, apple cider vinegar, and you will think you are winning the battle, but as soon as you give the yeast overgrowth some food again, e.g., sugars, mouldy cheese, mushrooms, wine, etc, it will grow back very quickly.

But if you take away the intolerance foods and heal the digestive tract, clean your kidneys, flush your liver, and recover your pancreas, the yeast overgrowth won't grow back, because the digestive tract can begin to function properly and at its optimum again, and will be re colonised, and a normal and balanced gut flora will be regained, keeping the bad bacteria in check.

Plain live or Bio yoghurt is a good supplement, as it contains lactobacillus, burglarious, and streptococcus lactis, these are extremely helpful in regaining good gut flora.

Notice I say PLAIN LIVE or BIO YOGHURT; this is because if you buy fruit yoghurts then automatically they will contain elements such as sugar, which will feed the bad bacteria, and affect your digestive system and the balance of good and bad bacteria.

Plain Live or Bio yoghurt should not affect you if you stay on the advised recovery programme, unless you are extremely food intolerant.

This is because there is no lactose (milk sugar) in live yoghurt, which will feed your yeast overgrowth; it has been converted into lactic acid by the live yoghurt making process.

Lactic acid also aids in neutralising elements produced when gluten or gliadin is present in the gut, gliadin is the fraction of wheat that most celiacs and wheat intolerants react to, so if you eat live yoghurt it usually neutralises any reactions to wheat, but only if the wheat has been eaten in small amounts, this often happens if you go out for a meal and accidentally eat some wheat.

Many celiacs have no reaction to small amounts of wheat if lactic acid from live yoghurt is eaten at the same time as the wheat.

Although I would not recommend you to eat wheat in recovery, even in small amounts, and not until all the liver flushes and kidney cleanses required to recover your system have been completed.

Plain Live or Bio plain yoghurt is not only very beneficial to restoring gut flora, it is also effective in reducing some vaginal infections such as Thrush (Trichomonas Vaginalis) in women, But do not have too much, one serving every day is enough at first to help maintain good gut flora, any more could give you loose bowels.

Some people find they can't even have Plain live or Bio yoghurt in the early stages of recovery, for about the first two months, so you will have to try it in the early stages, and gauge the reaction for yourself. If you cannot cope with the live yoghurt then take pre and pro biotics instead, as directed by your local health shop.

So to eradicate yeast overgrowth is very difficult, you have to be very strict with yourself, and not eat any of the foods listed at the end of this chapter, and only eat small amounts of the foods carrying this symbol # on the list of "foods that can be eaten" on pages 48-49, or the cut out wall chart on page 15, and commit yourself to some gallbladder and liver flushes, and the kidney cleanses.

KILLING OFF YEAST OVERGROWTH

You can use products such as Coconut milk, onions, garlic, apple cider vinegar, oregano or propolis to kill off the overgrowth, but don't take any of these for a period of 1 month or so after starting the diet, or the reaction could be very intense, and your system will not cope with the toxins produced by the dying yeast overgrowth, this will make you feel ill and tired.

So, start off with very small amounts of these and I mean very small amounts, if it is in liquid form, such as apple cider vinegar 1 teaspoon a day to start off with.

If you feel ill or get diarrhoea, stop for a few days and start again very slowly.

Propolis is good for killing off yeast overgrowth, but if you can eat onions or garlic and they don't make you ill then you will not need to take propolis, because the onions and or garlic will kill the yeast overgrowth just as efficiently as the propolis, plus it's one less supplement to remember to take, and the propolis can be quite expensive to buy, so you can save money as well.

I would also recommend you take the elements as discussed in the "vitamins and minerals" chapter starting on page 202, or refer to "the recovery programme chapter" on page 77, titled the second month of recovery, this will also help you detoxify better, but only take these as recommended.

Coconuts help because they contain Caprylic acid, this is toxic to many yeast infections, this will help to eradicate the overgrowth in the lower digestive tract, so drink some coconut milk, or eat a coconut on a regular basis.

I found in my case that it took 18 months or so to seriously get the overgrowth under control, and found in the latter stages that I had a sore throat and sore nasal passages for a time, and I partially lost my voice for a short time. I can only think that this must be the air passages, tonsils, and detoxification processes, related to your immune system in your throat recovering normality. Or the possibility that it may be the thyroid recovering.

You will require a series of gallbladder and liver flushes and the kidney cleanses to recover your system fully, after which you will find the yeast overgrowth will die back much faster, because your bile, pancreatic enzyme and hormone production will improve and re balance your PH (bowel acidity) and gut flora, as discussed in the, "What happens to the digestive tract chapter", starting on page 100.

A gallbladder and liver flush is highly recommended, indeed essential, if you have very bad yeast overgrowth, because this is yet another sign that your liver is at the very least clogged, and you may also have gallstones.

It's a long hard and difficult battle, but it seems that you cannot eradicate this with any speed; diligence is the name of the game.

The yeast overgrowth begins to die off naturally, albeit very slowly once the intolerance foods are taken away, this is obviously due to the recovery of the digestive tract, and stabilisation of digestive PH, but ingestion of the foods to be avoided in the list at the end of this chapter, keeps feeding the yeast overgrowth or Candida, and progress would be extremely slow without the exclusion of these products.

Once on the diet you may take a teaspoon of Apple cider vinegar in a mug of water, take this every other day for about two weeks, this will aid in killing off the yeast overgrowth.

Its important to stay on this advised diet, and not drink any sweet drinks as advised in the "what can I drink" chapter starting on page 70, for up to 2 years, to eradicate the yeast overgrowth fully.

Two years without a soft drink I hear you cry.

Sodium bicarbonate may be taken to kill off yeast overgrowth, but only after you have adopted the recovery diet, and completed some gallbladder and liver flushes, in most cases gut flora will stabilise and kill the yeast overgrowth once liver and pancreatic function have recovered, this should only be used in very small quantities, (half a teaspoon every other day), in some cases it is necessary to stabilise gut flora again.

Believe me if you think you are going to eradicate it in a couple of months, then you are dreaming, it may have taken you forty years to get into the condition you are in now, and therefore you obviously will not recover overnight.

AIDS TO KILLING YEAST OVERGROWTH

- Herbs (consult a naturopathic doctor or herbalist), they can be very beneficial.

- Coconut milk

- Cranberries, which can be quite bitter, but NOT cranberry juice, (cranberry juice is potentially very sweet, and feeds digestive yeast and bacterial overgrowth in your digestive tract, so you must remember, only cranberries, and not cranberry juice), eating cranberries is also very beneficial for thrush in women.

- They can be difficult to source, but many supermarkets do stock them on a seasonal basis.

- Garlic

- Onions

- Oregano

- Propolis

- Gallbladder and liver flushes, (by far the most important factor)

- Kidney treatments, (again very important)

- Bicarbonate of soda, (very small amounts, half a teaspoon every other day, and only after three or four gallbladder and liver flushes)

- Apple cider vinegar. (teaspoon a day, after one month on diet)

FOODS TO BE AVOIDED WITH YEAST OVERGROWTH

- Anything with refined sugar in it

- Anything fungusey (such as mushrooms)

- Anything yeasty (you are unlikely to come across yeast, because of the diet you will be following in this book, regarding the wheat, dairy etc, intolerance)

- Wine

- Grapes

- Raisins

- Sultanas

- Strawberries

- Tinned fruits in syrup

- Plums

- Mouldy cheeses (but you may have small quantities of goats cheese, or cottage cheese whilst in recovery)

- Mushrooms

If in doubt refer to this symbol -• on pages 48-49 or refer to the cut out wall chart on page 15.

Note
(Yeast overgrowth can also be a mechanical problem, caused after medical intervention, where a blind loop causes food to stagnate in the intestine, like a stagnant pond. Other illnesses may cause this condition, but in this book I am concerned with yeast overgrowth, in relation to food Intolerance)

ATHLETES FOOT, THICK TOENAILS, BACTERIA

People who are very intolerant usually have or have had Athletes foot, and often thick toenails as well as yeast overgrowth.

There is a definite connection with the yeast overgrowth on the tongue, the common connection is the lack of ability to absorb all the elements required to enable your immune and lymphatic system, to eliminate the bacteria or fungus that allows the athletes foot (Tinea Pedis) thick toenails to proliferate.

The correct acidity of sebum (skin secretions) and the correct chemical make up of skin secretions leaves us unable to kill off yeast and fungus on the skin and, especially on the toenails, and inside of toes, or folds of skin.
There are many fungi that can affect your nails Trychophyton Mentagrophytes, and Trychophyton Rubrum, are two of the more common fungi.

If you have very bad athletes foot or thick toenails you can relieve the symptoms dramatically, by taking two or three caps full of Apple cider vinegar, and putting it in a bowl of warm water, bathe your feet in this for about twenty minutes, do this for about four alternate nights.

This treatment will kill off the infections, but I have to say that it will slowly return if you do not change your diet, and complete any necessary gallbladder and liver flushes.

Treating these fungal conditions from the outside in, as in creams etc, is only masking the problem and not eradicating the fungi but controlling it. In most cases once you take away the ointment or cream the fungus begins to regroup, and your symptoms will return, especially if your feet become warm and damp.

Bacteria can also invade the body when you become food intolerant; some of the more common ones are Streptococcus pyogenes, Staphylococcus aureus, Pseudamonas aeruginosa, Escherichia coli, Propionibacterium acnes and Mycobacterium vaginalis.

You will probably not know if you have any of these invading bacterium, but if you have, they will begin to die back, and will ease once you begin the recovery programme.

It usually requires a series of gallbladder and liver flushes before your immune system can again begin to eradicate, or control these invaders of the body, and relieve you of these stubborn parasites.

Herbs can be extremely beneficial in helping to eradicate athlete's foot and fungal infections, but you must consult a professional herbalist or Naturopathic Doctor if you are to use them.

DO NOT self medicate by buying products from your local health shop; you may upset your digestive tract and impede recovery.

ACKNOWLEDGMENT

24th March 2004

Dear John,

Little did I know what on earth was wrong with me after Doctors continuously telling me "there is nothing wrong with me", untill after seeing a young women (Jane your sister) putting all these healthier foods into her basket at the supermarket, after asking her "was it for a perticular reason" or did she just like them. Her story about how her brother had researched long & hard to find an answer to his own Ill health, & many others, I was more than interested, as my intolerance to a whole range of food & drink was far to much to bear, after getting your book "are we intolerant to what WHEAT" & following its advice on food, what to eat & what not, and also the Kidney cleanse & gall bladder & liver flushes, I am improving leaps & bounds no more heart burn, or headaches, no more white spots appearing on my face, I am rarely exhausted anymore, my toiletry habits are back to normal, I feel 75% better all round & shall continue following the book till I am 100% and even after that, and hope others will see how well I have become & follow in my foot steps.

With my most sincere and heartfelt thanks I write this letter to you John...

you have made possible what Doctors have not.

Many Many Thanks
Pat Colgan

TOXINS AND OXIDANTS

WHICH PRODUCTS ARE TOXIC AND OXIDISING?

Every day your body is infiltrated by toxins and oxidants.

You may not realise that some things you come into contact with are toxins or oxidants, the following will give you some idea of what is toxic, and what is an oxidising.

Even the fumes from plastic wrappings on food products or plastic bottles, these may only have a small effect on the body, but nevertheless they are still toxins and have an effect, just because you don't notice the effect doesn't mean there isn't one.

Try cutting an onion in half and then wrap it in clingfilm for a week, and then notice that when you unwrap it, that the onion is far less pungent and intense, and that some of the potency of the onion has been imparted into the clingfilm, and the clingfilm has been imparted into the onion. The onion will actually taste of clingfilm, and the onion will have lost its potency, and taste of plastic.

Just to show you what I mean by oxidants, leave a pat of butter out on your worktop for some time, and watch the atmosphere start to break down the butter. This is the air oxidising it and breaking it down.

This is what oxidants try to do to your body tissue every day.

If you are fit and healthy your body can repair this damage without a problem, unless you overload your system, or some other force comes into play such as gained intolerance to wheat and dairy products. Your system then has too much to do and over the years begins to break down.

It loses some of its ability to repair all the damage done by the toxins and oxidants .Your digestive tract will degrade to the point where it almost treats wheat and dairy products as a toxin, and tries to flush them through your digestive system.

The dairy products also produce some toxins in your digestive tract, along with the wheat, this is yet another important reason for staying off wheat and dairy products, until you are well into recovery.

FRIED FOODS

Lets look at fried foods, if you fry anything in fat that is too hot, you are in effect burning it, and this produces oxidants, so potentially fish and chips are oxidants, or a fry up is oxidising, this tries to break down tissue.

So if you fry anything it is important not to have the fat too hot, this will burn the food, if you have the fat just hot enough to fry the food, and not burn it, this is all right, and will not produce masses of oxidants.

So if we want to repair the digestive system we can't eat, over fried food, or over cooked food that is burnt, But don't be too wary of fried food, the odd plate of chips now and then are all right; after all we need to let go now and then.

COFFEE

Coffee is an oxidant because it has been burnt to produce the beans. Anything burnt is an oxidant. Coffee is thought to be related to stomach cancer if drunk in large amounts, coffee also contains caffeine.

You wouldn't do it, but if you drank 200 cups of strong coffee in 1 day, the caffeine would kill you, so bear in mind that if you are a coffee addict and drink lets say 10 cups a day, you're on dangerous ground, whereas 1 cup a day would pause no problem at all, unless you have food intolerance, then it should be avoided all together in the early stages of recovery.

SMOKING

Smoking is about the worst thing you can do. This not only introduces lots of toxins and oxidisers into the system, but stops the system absorbing up to 60% of the vitamin C you intake, which is essential for repairing tissue or helping to neutralisie cancerous causing toxins and oxidants.

Smoking introduces lots of toxins into the entire body, of which I could list in abundance, to say the least smoking is like playing Russian roulette, especially if you are on a bad diet or have intolerance. It usually kills you in the end. Very few people live to a ripe old age and smoke.

ALCOHOL

Alcohol is a toxin and if taken in large quantities destroys the liver and damages many other organs. If you go out and drink a lot of alcohol at one go, "binge drinking", and you drank 14 units, that's the equivalent of 7 pints of average beer, or 5 bottles of stronger beer, then it will hinder your liver and pancreas in their production of bile and enzymes for about 10 days after, this means it will take your liver and pancreas 10 days to get back to where they were before you had the drink.

So if you go out drinking, and especially binge drinking on a weekly basis, you are damaging your liver and pancreas, and slowly degrading them. Until eventually you could develop diseases like, diabetes or pancreatitis, or liver damage, cirrhosis of the liver, your enzyme and bile production will almost certainly be impaired, thus you will not break down foods properly, you will begin to malabsorb leading to other deficiencies, and eventually possible digestive tract problems.

If you do go out binge drinking, then you will have noticed how you are slightly weak and tired for a few days after. This is your system trying to expel the toxins that have piled up in the system, it will also have affected your ability to break down foods, and affected your absorption pattern for a few days, its little wonder you feel slightly off for a few days.

To show you how the body can detoxify faster, try eating some Brussels sprouts, cauliflower, cabbage, or asparagus before you go out drinking and notice how much faster your body detoxifies and how much better you feel in the morning. This is due to the glucosinolates and homosacharides in these vegetables, they help you to expel alcohol at a much faster rate, if you drink slowly you wont even notice the effects of the alcohol. What these green foods do is to bolster your liver and kidneys ability to expel toxins, and help to heal the digestive tract.

This does not mean you can go out and drink; you shouldn't drink any alcohol at all, or at least very little, whilst we are trying to repair your digestive tract, and related organs.

I have experimented with these foods and it works, so when mummy said eat your greens she was right.

SUNLIGHT

Sunlight can damage your skin, but in general is very beneficial to your body, it helps to heal wounds, kills microbes and bacteria, and when sunlight falls on your skin a reaction takes place and you convert 7dehydrocholesterol from the sunlight into vitamin D, which in turn helps you to process calcium, but if you get too much sun it can cause damage, as we all know, and can begin to damage your epidermis and destroy your skin, and in the extreme lead to skin cancer.

FUMES

The fumes produced by anything burning are an oxidant or toxin.

So barbecued foods, fried foods, car fumes, paint fumes, cleaners, detergents, sprays, washing up liquid, man made oils, any smoke, alcohol, coffee, you could name many more are all toxins or oxidisers.

So if you want to fill your body with toxins and oxidisers have a barbecue, with burnt food, next to a busy road, in the middle of a city, whilst smoking and drinking alcohol and coffee, without any clothes on, on the sunniest day of the year, oh and don't forget to do some painting at the same time, then clear the air with an aerosol spray of some kind, that little combination should kill you off pretty quick.

Scary stuff ey, but its true, toxins and oxidants are all around us every day, and if you think your body has gained the ability to cope with these modern toxins and oxidants, and keep coping with them, in the little time they have been around, then you are deluding yourself.

It takes hundreds, even thousands of years for your body to even think about adapting to these modern toxins and oxidants, let alone the few decades our bodies have been exposed to them.

Even our recent descendants did not have the same barrage of oxidisers and toxins, that we have every day, from even ordinary everyday products such as cleaners, car fumes, sprays, paints, oils, plastics, washing up liquid, etc, etc.

Well lets not get carried away, your body has an amazing ability to cope with these products if you are fit and healthy, but couple this with food intolerance and the bodily function begins to collapse, and its then that we begin to spiral into the abyss, and descend down the symptoms chain.

Be aware that poor diet, over cooked fried fast foods, and smoking and drinking in the main, are the initiating factor in many digestive failures, couple this with gained food intolerance and a clogged liver due to a lifelong bad diet, and we have an even more serious problem.

Natural and neutral foods, are the thing to eat once you have gained food intolerance, especially fruits and vegetables, as they contain natural enzymes, which help to break themselves down once in the body, and help detoxification and the expulsion of foreign substances, some oil and fats are also required to aid in this process, but you can eat friendly oils such as olive oil, and fish oils.

Anything processed is much harder for the body to break down, and puts stress on your digestive tract, many of these processed foods contain toxins, oxidisers, and preservatives, your digestive tract has to unravel the preservatives before it can begin to break down the foods you are eating, so stay away from them, only eat natural unprocessed foods. The easiest way to advise you is to say, don't eat anything in a package or tin.

You must eat the low toxin foods as recommended on the "foods that can be eaten" list on pages 48-49, or refer to the cut out wall chart on page 15, then your system has very little to detoxify.

If you are in the depths of intolerance an overload of toxins will leave you tired, so it's essential to keep away from the toxins, if we are going to recover from the long standing, and slowly gained food intolerance, due to the degradation of the digestive tract.

All these things have been degrading your system for years, so we have to rebuild it, which we try to do using the recovery programme and the foods that can be eaten whilst in recovery.

TOXIC OVERLOAD

The main reason why potentially fatal conditions, such as cancer, are becoming more and more common is because most of the population are on such a bad diet, and are also coming into contact with many of the aforementioned chemicals.

Our modern diet fills our system with toxins and oxidants, every day. Problems begin to arise, because you're lymphatic and immune (detoxification system), can only expel and eradicate these toxins and oxidants, at a rate equal to the fitness of your detoxification system.

If your detoxification system is sluggish, and you are ingesting foods that are full of toxins and oxidants, due to poor diet, and you add this to being exposed to many everyday toxic elements in sprays etc, and you also smoke and drink, you could be eradicating toxins and oxidants more slowly than you are taking them in, if this is the case then you are deemed to be in what I call "toxic overload".

If this scenario occurs, you will be in a dangerous situation. Many intolerants say to me, "it's hard to explain, I feel like I am being poisoned or something, I feel sort of ill". They are in toxic overload, and wide open to many illnesses and even cancer.

If these conditions persist for many years they can damage DNA in cells and potentially initiate proliferation of defective cell production, these defective cells may be cancerous.

This is another reason why I put you on the diet, and recovery programme. The diet is very low in toxins and oxidants; therefore even if your detoxification system is running at a low level, it should be able to eradicate any toxins that the advised friendly diet contains. This will bring you well below your toxic overload threshold, and you will begin to feel much better within two or three weeks.

People often report having a headache and slight stomach upset when they first start the diet, this is a good indication that they have been in toxic overload.

Their system and many bodily functions are switching back from toxic overload, to toxic underload, they may be in toxic underload for the first time in many years, and therefore will be eradicating toxins faster than they are taking them in, this is why many report a vast improvement in their well being, after as little as two or three weeks on the diet and recovery programme.

SENSITIVITY TO TOXINS AND OXIDANTS

The more food intolerant you are and the more you will react to exposure to oxidants and especially toxins. Your immune and lymphatic system will be very sluggish if you become very food intolerant, therefore your ability to expel toxins and oxidants will be very much reduced, so extreme intolerants cannot cope with any addition to the toxic load from an outside source such as car fumes, paint fumes, pollen, moulds etc.

This is because of the lack of ability to break down, extract, absorb and interact all the elements from the food you eat, you will not have the elements required to run your immune, detoxification and lymphatic system properly, and therefore you will begin to loose the ability to tolerate some irritants such as car fumes, paint fumes, pollen, moulds etc, your system cannot identify them, and eradicate them, so often there is an intense reaction.

Even a very small exposure to some substances such as car fumes, or dust, or even some foods, can in many extreme intolerants cause quite strong reactions, such as sore nasal passages, a sore or hot feeling on the tongue, a skin rash, dry patches of skin or sore skin could be the reaction, or a feeling of being filled with flu can often be the response.

It is not possible to predict which substances may cause a reaction.

It depends how far down the intolerance chain you have fallen, people who are in the early stages of intolerance with a low score on the symptoms list on pages 18 to 21, don't tend to notice or be affected by or have any response to irritants.

But the further you fall into the depths of intolerance, the more you will become sensitive to many irritating products which could range from, foods, gasses, smoke, pollen, perfume, paint, detergents, even rubber or plastic can cause a reactive response to extreme intolerants.

The good news is that if you adopt the recovery programme and diet detailed in this book, and flush and clean the liver, and kidneys, you will slowly regain the ability to extract all the elements from the food you eat and therefore your detoxification, immune, and lymphatic system, will have all the nutrients and elements they require to identify and control these irritants, without overreacting, your body will begin to regain the ability to cope with infiltration of these irritating substances and eradicate them, with little or no reaction at all.

You will have dramatically increased you toxic load threshold, and therefore be able to cope with infiltration of many foreign substances with no reaction, but a word of warning, do not go back to your old eating and drinking habits, or after a few years you will drift back into the mire of food intolerance.

Some people do retain a reactive immune response to certain substances even after full recovery, this is due to their immune system being activated in the past, triggering the production of cells that will always recognise the offending elements, these cells may lie dormant for years, but when they encounter the offending element again they will respond, causing rashes, burning, soreness etc.

TIME, MEMORY, STRESS AND THE MIND

TIME

Elderly people used to tell me that time will go much faster as you get older, and this is generally true, but I now know that the state of your health has an important bearing on your perception of time.

A week used to zip by when I was in the depths of my intolerance.

But after recovery I have definitely observed that time appears to go much slower, now after recovery a week seems to last much longer, and you will become much more in touch with your environment, and more aware, and alert, and not cocooned in the world your head used to live in.

MEMORY AND THE MIND

This is another definite observation, arrived at after working with many food intolerants, virtually everyone reported dramatic improvements after recovery, especially in their name memory.

When you are in the depths of intolerance, your name memory may be effected dramatically, and you may even find yourself forgetting the names of people you see on a regular basis.

This can be extremely embarrassing, and if you are talking with friends you tend to listen for their name to crop up in the conversation, and try and put it firmly back in your memory.

Sometimes you can even forget what you are talking about, right in the middle of a conversation, you just loose your train of thought.

You may find it hard to concentrate for long periods of time, and if you are doing some secretarial task, which involves memory, you will find it very hard to keep concentration.

My most embarrassing moment was when a hotel receptionist asked the names of my three daughters, I remembered two of them, Kirsty and Sophie, and then proceeded to take about thirty seconds, each of which seemed like an eternity, to search my mind and remember the name of my third daughter Charlotte. I felt like a right plonker I can tell you. Thank god that sort of memory loss doesn't happen any more.

Once you have fully recovered, there is a definite and noticeable improvement in your short term, and name memory.

Even logical rational thought can be impaired, if you have a worrying problem your mind scurries around in a repeating and anxiety driven jumble of thoughts, an answer could be arrived at, and then you will repeat the thoughts again, and arrive at the same answer. This however may not content your mind, and again and again you will work out the same scenario, until your mind is at a point where it will begrudgingly accept the inevitable conclusion and answer.

This reaction is anxiety based, and after recovery you will find your mind more contented, and less stressed by a problem, you will definitely worry less and be far less anxious.

I find many people with this condition who run their own business, these people often worry excessively to the point of becoming depressed, as they advance further into food intolerance everything begins to get on top of them, and they have a feeling of despair.

Even when things are running relatively well, their mind is not contented after analysing a situation, and the subject they are worrying about will not go away, it keeps preying on their mind. These scenarios have the potential to lead on to depression and in the extreme, even self-harm consequences, potentially suicide.

Every person who has fully recovered from intolerance always report the same, they say they do not become stressed over problems at work, they are able to take things in their stride, even a serious problem is analysed in the mind, and an answer is arrived at and that is that, their mind is content with the answer, if something very serious happens they can deal with it, without getting slightly panicky, it almost becomes an enjoyable challenge, instead of an unmitigated disaster of epic proportions, which is insurmountable.

These people again find an inner peace and a willingness to accept events as they are, and not let small problems dominate their lives.

I myself experienced the previously described patterns of thought and worried continually over small problems, I made mountains out of molehills, it is very difficult to explain to someone who has never experienced worry and deep anxiety, how your way of thinking changes after full recovery.

You mind will change the way it views a problem, the best way I can describe it is to say, now the inevitable conclusion to a given problem is acceptable to the mind, whereas before the inevitable conclusion was not acceptable to the mind.

I do not know exactly why the brain recovers it's thought patterns in this way, I can only think that after full recovery it is being fully nourished, and therefore functions correctly, or more likely the correct chemical balance is regained, there is also a strong possibility that there are less toxins entering the brain.

This is yet another observation after working with many recovered food intolerants, for anyone who has experienced these depressive states, it is the release from trauma and stress, which makes life so much easier.

I was amazed to find that it was not just myself that found this phenomena but virtually all the people who had fully recovered, so it was a fantastic secondary discovery and realisation, only realised and discovered after myself and others had fully recovered, it was unexpected and unpredicted, but is one of the most important aspects of regained health when you are full recovery.

STRESS AND THE COMMON BILE DUCT

It is often said that stress causes stomach disorders, this is a broad statement and often used in very loose terms to explain stomach and bowel problems, often IBS.

This statement is at best only partially true, stress alone does not cause stomach and bowel disorders.

The instant that you begin to loose the ability to break down some of the foods you eat, is the instant that you will begin to loose the ability to extract all the nutrients your brain requires to function properly, you will slowly begin to become more anxious, and less able to cope with a heavy workload, you will become more stressed, what was once a minor problem may begin to prey on your mind.

But importantly it is not the stress that is, or has, initiated your stomach problems, the stress factor only comes into play after the liver becomes partially blocked and you loose some of your ability to break down food, the lack of absorption of nutrients then decreases the brains ability to cope with problems, this leads to anxiety, and if you work or live in a tense or stressful environment, muscle tension.

You are already an intolerant teetering on the edge of advanced intolerance.

This stressed state can often be the straw that breaks the camels back, when related to the digestive tract.

Why?

Because it can partially contribute to an even more reduced ability to freely pass bile enzymes and hormones down the common bile duct, tipping you over the edge into advanced intolerance.

As you become more stressed your muscles tend to tighten slightly, even the muscles within your digestive tract will react in this way, therefore the muscles controlling the valve work within the stomach, and more importantly the muscles controlling the common bile duct can begin to tense up and contract slightly, this will impair the free flow of bile enzymes and hormones even more, and therefore you will further impede your ability to break down food properly.

Because of the reduced ability to break down foods peristalsis will also be slightly affected, and therefore the passage of food throughout your digestive tract will be affected.

So stress can have an effect on the digestive tract, but only after breakdown and absorption problems have depleted nutrient extraction and absorption, and starved the brain of vital nutrients, it is only then that the previously mentioned scenarios within the common bile duct and digestive tract come into play, and part of the reason why advanced food intolerants are often made worse if in a continually stressful environment.

Stress is only compounding the problem in some people, but only a small percentage of intolerants are in a very stressful environment; remember stress is not the cause of your digestive problems, don't let a doctor tell you that stress is the cause of your problems, or it's all in your head, it is definitely not the cause of your problems, it may only ever be a contributory factor.

THE DIGESTIVE TRACT AND THE MIND

Patently memory and brain function are affected by the ingestion of the intolerance foods, or should I say by the lack of nutrients the brain requires to work efficiently, due to the lost abilities within your digestive tract.

Your brain will also have been filled with toxins, due to inefficiencies in the blood brain barrier (astrocytes), this will further reduce its function; this again is due to your digestive problems.

Therefore it stands to reason that there is a distinct possibility that brain function is affecting or changing the workings of the body.

Many people who are sent home after tests at their local hospital, and told that they must try and relax you're not really ill, or that half your problem is in your head, are actually in a way being told the truth, but and this is an important but, the doctor is inferring that your medical condition, often IBS, is caused by the way you think, whereas what I am saying, is that your digestive tract condition is being controlled by the fact that your mind is running your digestive tract at a different level, and trying to compensate and keep the digestive tract at a level where it can still extract elements, but expel the intolerance foods.

All these complications are as a result of ingesting the foods you have become intolerant to, and the lack of ability to break them down and eradicate the toxins they produce; these conditions are not being initialised by the brain.

If brain function is affecting the bodily function then the brain has first been degraded, and/or is trying to aid the digestive tract in coping with infiltration by some foreign body, in this case your gained intolerance to food.

Therefore we have a vicious circle where the body initially becomes intolerant to certain foods, and looses the ability to break them down and extract vital nutrients, and this very slowly over the years degrades internal organs and deprives the brain, then the brain especially the memory does not function properly.

Your mind tries to change slightly some of your digestive functions, it's trying to control the crisis in your digestive tract and keep you going, it's trying to alleviate your many symptoms on pages 18 to 21, Its not the brain causing the problem, the brain is trying to stabilise the digestive tract.

Whilst these conditions exist it only takes a slight upset to tip the balance, and give say someone with irritable bowel disease (IBS), diarrhoea.

Lets take a normal healthy person is put them a nervous situation, a job interview or a stage appearance, notice I say a nervous situation and not a stressful situation, then this normal healthy person may experience slight loose bowels, or butterflies in the stomach, this would be considered a normal reaction.

Now lets put someone with food intolerance, irritable bowel or chronic fatigue in the same nervous situation, they will appear to have a severe reaction, but in reality they are having the same reaction as a healthy person, they are just starting from a different point, they are on the very edge of diarrhoea or stomach and bowel reactions already, because or their food intolerance, and these nervous situations take them far deeper into these reactive states than a normal healthy person, nerves cause the bowel to expel its contents.

Again it's not the brain causing the problem, but the brains normal response to a situation, on top of what is already a delicate situation caused by gained food intolerance.

After a few visits to the doctors with stomach upset, and possibly after having various tests, there is often no measurable definable illness found, and therefore the doctor could assume that their stomach upset is anxiety driven and is relatively normal, and so often all that are prescribed are antacids, or you are told that there is nothing wrong with you, go home and relax and stop worrying, its your nerves upsetting your system.

You may be told many people are like you at your age, your getting older, or you could be told there is a possibility you could have slight irritable bowel symptoms.

If you have some unexplained long standing digestive problem, then I say to you that there is a very strong possibility, that its more likely that you have gained food intolerance to something your ingesting, rather than a nervous, stress or worry related problem.

So the underlying problem is being completely missed by many doctors, because it is not measurable definable or obvious, it just cannot be that half the nation feels " not quite right" most of the time, patently its not the mind causing the problem, another force is at work, and mainly its what we are eating in our modern diet, and the consequential problems that develop through a lifetime of over indulgence in these products.

Another factor related to stress and digestion is what is referred to as the "fight or flight" response, this directly influences digestive activity, our modern society and the pressures that are put on many of us each day, can directly affect digestion, if you are in an excessively stressful job, then you may be tipped into the "fight or flight" syndrome, where your body changes the way it functions.

Historically you would only be tipped into this situation if you were terrified by a growling lion, or other such terror, where you would be required to run in fear (flight), or stop and fight for your life (fight), under these circumstances your digestion is almost completely turned off, and your bodily functions relating to muscles and the release of energy are turned up, after all you don't need digestion if you think you are about to die, but you do need as much energy as possible to run and escape or fight for your life.

Some people are in such a stressful job, that they can be tipped into fight or flight just through going to work, this phenomena I have seen in healthy fit people without food intolerance, and therefore should not be confused with food intolerance gained through liver and pancreatic dysfunction.

This is quite an interesting thought, if we all ate a much better diet, and flushed our livers and flushed our kidneys, then in theory the collective thought and intelligence of the nation could be elevated to a higher plane, would this make us a superior race? Behave John, now you're getting carried away.

FOOD AND THE MIND

Once you have fully recovered your digestive tract will be functioning properly, and extracting and utilising all the vitamins, minerals, and nutrients necessary to run your entire body at its full potential, therefore your brain will switch off the hunger pangs, the neurons will stop firing, and your body will have all the ingredients it requires.

Your body knows when it has enough of one or other elements required to run efficiently.

A good example to try and explain this, is to look at the reactions of small children to food.

Small children will often push aside food after eating a good amount of lets say, a first course, they may say I am full, but put something sweet in front of them, lets say peaches and ice cream, and they will very quickly change their mind.

In truth, when these children do this, they are not necessarily making a totally conscious decision to reject the first course or the food they have just been eating, they are very sensitive to the ingestion of nutrients and to a degree their mind knows when they have had enough of the elements in the food they have just eaten in the first course, the neurons stop firing and they genuinely could actually feel full of those nutrients or at least satisfied.

But when they get sight and smell of the peaches or ice cream to a degree the neurons begin to fire again and tell them they are hungry again.

Young children are extremely sensitive in this area, and you will find that after recovery you too will begin to feel satisfied after eating lets say lots of vegetables or a main course, and your hunger will turn off, but if you smell something different from a/or the food you have just eaten a lot of, your hunger pangs will turn on again, to a degree your brain knows when it requires these varying nutrients.

After full recovery your body will be very quick to respond and will become very sensitive if it smells and sees something it knows it is short of. It's not actually just as simple as the previously explained, a combination of factors involving smell, taste, sight, past experience and the efficiency of your digestive tract that are responsible and necessary for these senses to return.

In food intolerants the duodenum and jejunum are not extracting nutrients, or vitamins and minerals properly in early recovery, so you will be constantly short of these vitamins and minerals, it just so happens that many of the nutrients that the duodenum and jejunum extract are found in bread, little wonder you almost become addicted to it, your mind is always looking for these nutrients, typically, thiamine, niacin, and riboflavin, your hypothalamus in your brain, tells you that you are short of these nutrients, and switches the hunger pangs on, often making you feel hungry all the time.

This is why some people often say to me, I am virtually addicted to bread and find it very difficult to give it up, they have not been extracting the nutrients from the bread and so every time they smell it the neurons begin to fire, and they feel hungry, to a degree their mind knows it requires these nutrients, so again the only way to remedy this situation is to clean the digestive tract, liver and kidneys, and make them function efficiently again.

Take my word for it, you will find these scenarios begin to re assert themselves once full recovery has been attained, you will begin to notice your hunger pangs turning on and off again as they did when you were a child.

Your mind communicates with your digestive tract and your digestive tract communicates with your mind.

N.B
In this chapter I am dealing with the mind in relation to intolerance of foods.

Obviously other conditions also exist and can affect the way people react around food, such as Bolemia, Anorexia.

In some people there is a different reaction to the one described above. These people may have suffered a traumatic event at some stage in their early life.

This can have an effect on the digestive tract long term, even without intolerance to foods or a clogged liver, this condition is rare and difficult to diagnose, and can involve psychiatry to uncover the causal factor or factors, therefore we won't go any further into this type of digestive upset.

THE COLD PHENOMENA

When you are in the depths of food intolerance, you seem to need a lot of heat to keep you warm, especially if you are sat doing nothing, but soon overheat when doing exercise.

Your thermostat seems not to be working properly.

It's like you're too hot on the inside and too cold on the outside, although you will be if your stomach is enflamed.

For some reason you may experience a short period, usually 3 to 6 months into recovery, where you feel very cold.

If it is summer you may not notice too much, but if it is winter you will definitely notice that you feel very cold for a period, and external limbs, fingers, toes, etc, will freeze if it is a cold day.

This seems to last for 2 to 3 months, you can wrap up as much as you want and still can't keep warm.
This happened to me and other people I have followed through recovery, many of us seem to go through this strange period.

Once you begin to recover your body seems to reverse, as it then starts to become warmer on the outside and cooler on the inside, so when you are inactive you still feel warm with little clothing on, even on a cool day.

Your thermostat seems to start working better; you don't overheat the same, or sweat as much when doing physical exercise.

I can only think this must be because the internal organs have had the intolerance foods taken away and initially the inflammation in the system goes down, so your internal temperature drops, but for a while you don't absorb properly so you don't have fuel to burn to keep you warm.

But the more you recover and absorb better, the more fuel you have to burn to keep you warm.
Of course there is a very good possibility that your circulation improves after eating the right foods, and taking a little exercise, therefore your extremities should be warmer anyway.

So the body seems to reverse from warmer inside and cooler outside to cooler inside and warmer outside.

Maybe there's nothing wrong with the bodies thermostat in that I can't prove this, but if you take the average temperature between the outside layers, as you would with a normal thermometer in the mouth or under the arm, then you are only taking an average position in the body to take a temperature, and internal organs of the body could be warmer than they should be, and the outside cooler than it should be, the trouble is that you can't easily take the temperature of an internal organ relative to an external organ, and therefore it would have to be done in a controlled environment.

Anyway enough theorising, this hot and cold phenomena is just an observation I thought I'd put in, its another indication and reaction in mid recovery.

A more detailed explanation of temperature regulation, and the possible causes of an inability to regulate body temperature efficiently, can be found on page 274 renin, angiotensinogen, ACE, and feeling cold.

AFTER FULL RECOVERY

You will find that after full recovery, your body will be much more able to keep your temperature stable.

If doing physical exercise you will find that you will still sweat, but it will not pour off you, as it may have done before, and you will be able to do quite a lot of exercise before you begin to sweat.

You will not experience excessive reactions to the hot and cold weather, if you are on holiday in a very hot country, others around you may complain that it is too hot, and you will think, well it doesn't feel that hot to me, but if you think back to before you made a full recovery, you will realise that you too used to find a lot of heat overpowering, making you tired and listless.

On the other hand if it is a very cold day, you will be warm enough without having to get well wrapped up to insulate you from the cold, you will not freeze as you did on cold days before you embarked on this recovery programme, and in the midst of recovery.

Your body will have regained its ability to cope within a wider band of hot and cold weather.

EXERCISE AND REST

EXERCISE

I know from experience that when you are recovering, too much exercise is as bad as too little, you can basically use more energy than you are producing.

In the case of chronic fatigue (ME), induced by food intolerance, you may not be able to exercise at all in the early stages of recovery. Some of these people can't even get to work without feeling exhausted, and consequently cannot hold down a job.

If in the early stages of recovery you use more energy than you are producing, this will leave you very tired and exhausted. Therefore it is very difficult to quantify the amount of exercise you can do, because the more you recover, the more exercise you can do without feeling exhausted.

So start slowly by doing short walks of maybe only a few hundred yards.

If you have chronic fatigue (ME), your body will tell you if you are using more energy than you are producing, and you will exhaust your system very quickly if you overdo it.

You need to do some exercise to keep your cardiovascular, lymphatic, and circulatory systems active and efficient, but don't try to cram it into some small gap in your day, this then becomes stressful and not beneficial, and will make you more tired.

If you exercise you take in oxygen which is vital for the repair of tissue amongst other things, if you exercise you will recover much faster, but be careful not to leave yourself exhausted, this is worse than no exercise at all in the early stages of recovery, as it leaves your body drained, because its not breaking down or absorbing nutrients properly.

If you look back thousands of years, you would not find man doing violent exercise for long periods or time, he would walk most of the time, up hill and down dale, this is good exercise.

He would run to catch prey, or take flight if in a frightening situation, but these would be short bursts and not prolonged violent exercise.

I have observed many people who take exercise three, four, or even five times a week to try and keep fit, and often this exercise is exhaustive, and very demanding. Often these people are eating the wrong diet and don't have a natural fitness and therefore find the exercise they do is hard work, these people are actually increasing the stress levels on their body, mentally as well as physically, their body is working at the limit all the time.

If you put someone on the correct diet they will slowly attain a natural bodily fitness over a few months, this person could be just as fit and healthy with very little exercise other than a good walk, once or twice a week, as the person who eats the wrong diet and takes intense exercise three four or five times a week.

I would go so far as to say that some people who take vast amounts of exercise are actually wasting their time, unless they adopt the correct diet, and are sure there digestive tract is fully functional.

After all if these people take all this exercise there should be lots of them living into extremely old age, this is definitely not the fact, by far the vast majority of these people live only slightly longer than someone on a relatively good diet, with an efficient digestive tract and little exercise.

You may have heard the story about Fred Bloggs, who ran 5 miles a day and died at the ripe old age of 55, at his funeral everyone was commenting and saying, "ooh poor Fred, "but wasn't he was fit when he died" ?.

I think the patently obvious question springs to mind. I wonder if Fred was OVERDOING IT AND ON THE WRONG DIET ?.

If you quiz many very old people who have never exercised on a regular basis, you inevitably find that they have in the most part eaten a good diet all their lives, although it may not have been a conscious decision on their part to adopt a healthy diet.

You usually find these people have lived a moderate life, everything in moderation, they will have had some exercise throughout their lives, but it was not a conscious decision on their part to keep them fit and healthy, it was only as part of their every day life, and participation in some social event, a Sunday walk for instance.

Bodily fitness begins in the first instance with diet, there is no way your body can perform properly with the wrong fuel and a clogged system.

In the early stages of recovery too much exercise = a drained system.

Therefore rest is as important as exercise.

Strong evidence is beginning to be uncovered by experiments on people who are trying to diet, that very short bursts of exercise, even 30 to 60 seconds of very violent, rapid exercise, four or five times a week, can be just as beneficial as jogging for hours.

Your muscles especially, carry a memory of the recent levels of exercise that you may have undertaken, if there are sufficient nutrients in your system, your muscles will replenish themselves, and build up to the level of strength required to undertake the previous level of exercise again.

If you are not extracting and absorbing nutrients properly from your digestive tract, then your muscles will be constantly short of energy, and you will feel weak, but your muscles will retain the memory of the level of activity you have previously undertaken, and will retain that memory for up to two weeks or so after the activity, sometimes people complete a gallbladder and liver flush, and within twelve hours they literally spring back to life and are full of energy, you may have had a sluggish liver for years, and if you suddenly unblock it, it is like turning a tap on, all of a sudden your muscles have the nutrients to work with, and build up to their recent memory level, many people find almost instant recovery after a series of liver flushes, they cannot believe that you can go from lethargy one day, to bounding energy the next.

REST

In these modern times there isn't much time for rest if you have a lifestyle like mine, but you have to change your lifestyle somehow. Although I know from my own experience that this is very difficult when you have a busy life.

You need as much rest as your body tells you. If you feel tired when you rise in the morning, then you have not had enough sleep or rest, although this situation will improve as you recover, and you will find you are less tired, and recover much faster after exercise as recovery continues.

This is hard to quantify, as some people need more sleep than others, but you will find that if you take away the intolerance foods, and eat the right foods you will quickly feel less tired, and when you do tire, it is a more natural tiredness, and a short nap will recharge your batteries, because your body is beginning to work at its optimum.

For instance I used to sleep for 8 to 10 hrs and be just as tired when I woke as when I went to bed, and also felt lethargic for an hour or so after rising, and have to have an hours sleep in the day as well, even then I was still tired and exhausted.

Now I find that 8hrs recharges my batteries and I may have a 10 to 20-minute power nap in the day, most days I don't even need the power nap, I now find this is all the sleep I need.

Feeling slightly tired is normal and different from the exhaustive tiredness you feel if you have chronic fatigue (ME), which prolonged food intolerance induces. There is what I call a natural tiredness, and then there is the exhaustive tiredness that is associated with chronic fatigue (ME). This you will understand once recovery begins to take place.

Natural tiredness is different from exhaustive tiredness: natural tiredness is a pleasant, woozy, naturally relaxed, and sleepy feeling, but exhaustive tiredness is an overwhelming uncontrollable feeling that you have to sleep or rest, its an unpleasant drained feeling, you may have disturbed sleep, and even wake up in your sleep feeling exhausted and tired with aching muscles, but cannot get back to sleep again even though you are feeling very tired, this exhaustive tiredness will begin to ease once recovery is under way.

Ideally you should try to go to bed before midnight, you produce many hormones at different times of the day, and some of these hormones regulate your waking and sleeping patterns, your sleep pattern, and the benefit you gain from sleep, is much improved if you go to bed at say 10 o'clock and rise at say 6.30, rather than go to bed at midnight and rise at 8.30. you will be working with your natural hormonal cycle, if you go to bed at 10 o'clock.

When you fly east or west on holiday you are interfering with your hormonal cycle, it can take up to two weeks for your hormones to reset themselves, so if you fly to America from Britain for two weeks holiday, your hormones have almost reset by the end of the holiday, then you come home and require another two weeks to reset fully again, this is commonly known as jetlag.

You will experience similar jetlag symptoms if you go to bed after ten o, clock ,and especially if you go to bed after midnight, that groggy feeling you get next morning is due to hormonal regulation imbalance.

People who go out and have a few drinks and come in after midnight feel groggy in the morning and put it down to the drink, but these people would have the same groggy feeling the next morning if they went to bed after midnight and did not have a drink.

Give yourself some quality time, for instance I never had time to sit and read a paper, but now I try and make time, it rests the body and takes you mind away from daily demands.

It's your life and your body. You owe it to yourself, you can't work all the time.

If you have a holiday don't try and crush too much into the week or two you have off, take time to relax and use the opportunity to rest. The world won't stop because you haven't done all those D.I.Y jobs, or visited all the theme parks.

I'm the worst one to give you this advice, I used to rush around all the time, and have to finish everything before I'd started, and take every job on that came along.

So try to get some control in your life, working like hell will only make you feel richer, materialistically speaking, not health-wise.

People that are happy with their lot, and take life at a steady pace tend to live longer! Think about it.

Take time to eat, and don't throw food down your throat to get back to the job in hand, this is stressful. And if you don't chew food properly, your chances of breaking it down and absorbing it properly are very much reduced.

Yes, I hear you say, it's easier said than done, but you owe it to yourself to do these things.

In this modern age most of us are too busy making a living to have quality time, so get control of your life, and don't let it control you. The company you work for won't collapse if you're not there, and you won't be, if with this food intolerance you carry on rushing around playing "chase the possessions".

You will inevitably find that as you recover you have more time anyway because you need less rest and sleep, and have more energy and feel more alive, believe me I've been there.

OBSERVATIONS

I now realise that in the past I never had the energy I have now, and that I had obviously had my food intolerance and clogged liver all my life.

Its nice to be able to do a days work without it absolutely draining me. I can now run a mile, or climb a steep hill or mountain with little effort, I have far less sleep, and have far more energy, and feel more alive, and more in touch and at one with my environment and surroundings.

So to sum up be careful when exercising and don't overdo it, even if 100 yards is too much at the start. Leave it for a week and try again. Let your body recover sufficiently first, to be fit you don't need to run two miles a day.

After full recovery a half hour walk or a run out on the bike, twice a week, over a good hill, is enough to get the heart pumping and keep you fit.

You don't have to perform like superman to be fit and healthy.

Natural health is attained through diet, not exercise.

So exercise and rest, and make sure you get good exercise and rest, again everything in moderation, as my grandma used to tell me.

VITAMINS AND MINERALS

Many people are being persuaded to take many vitamin and mineral substitutes as a result of advertising or hype, when there is nothing wrong with them, or certainly nothing that a slightly better diet wouldn't rectify.

I have found many people with food intolerance taking multivitamins and different concoctions, but they are only treating and alleviating symptoms and not confronting the causes of their condition, these drugs which is basically what they are, may make you feel slightly better but you are by no means well.

If your digestive tract is not functioning properly, especially your duodenum and jejunum, then you can take all the vitamin and mineral substitutes you like, but there is going to be very little absorption of these elements, you will not only be wasting your money, but often, actually compounding an already delicate situation within your digestive tract, and could actually be making your symptoms worse.

Many people take antacids, but anyone who takes a lot of antacids will hinder the absorption of vitamins and minerals, especially if they are taken over a lengthy period of time.

Many people are often prescribed the drug Colofax or anti depressants, the anti depressants especially are often used to try and relax the digestive tract, and also try and stabilise peristalsis, relieving symptoms, usually of I.B.S. But this is only relieving symptoms, and not addressing the causes of their problems.

Often if you go to a health shop they will prescribe a complementary or herbal remedy for digestive problems, but this again is only treating the symptoms and not addressing the causes, many digestive related drugs are only relieving symptoms, this is very serious because their underlying condition is still there, when it comes to the digestive tract we must stop treating symptoms, and address the cause or causes of the problem, starting with diet, and then cleansing your system.

Most people know very little or nothing at all about vitamin and mineral substitutes, with very little or no understanding at all, of what these elements are actually doing once in the body. For instance if you take vitamin E and Iron together both will be hindered, as one hinders the absorption of the other.

Another good example is vitamin C, if you eat plenty of fruit and vegetables you will get all the vitamin C your body needs, if you take in any more than the body requires it will go straight through you. This is because vitamin C it is very abundant in nature, your body has evolved without the need to create the facility or the ability to store it.

But if you look at vitamin E, which is not as abundant in nature, the body has had to evolve a system to store some of this in your liver; it then has a reserve to work with in lean times.

These scenarios are adopted by the body for many other vitamins and minerals, some are stored and some are not, dependant on historic availability in nature of the nutrient or mineral.

ANAEMIA

Some elements such as vitamin B12 are actually produced through interaction of elements within the digestive tract, little is obtained from your diet, especially the modern diet, although some can be obtained from liver, fish, or eggs, so as you can see if your gut flora is upset and your liver and pancreas don't function properly, and produce enough bile, enzymes, and hormones then you will not produce the conditions within the gut to manufacture vitamin B12.

The other problem with vitamin B12 is that you may produce some or supplement it but your intestine is not functioning correctly when you have gained food intolerance, therefore you may not absorb it properly at your terminal ileum, until you have recovered somewhat, in the extreme a lack of vitamin B12 can leave you with the more serious pernicious anaemia!

Vitamin B12 or iron deficiency can both lead to upset haemoglobin which can lead to the usual forms of anaemia, and the lack of oxygen carrying red blood cells, many intolerants have this type of anaemia before starting this recovery programme, that is why I often advocate you take iron in the early stages of recovery, as detailed in the recovery programme.

B12 and iron is vital for the nervous system, and replacement of cells.

Some iron is often required in the early stages of recovery, but do not take this on the same day as vitamin E, remember E hinders iron absorption, and iron hinders E absorption.

Iron requires a very high level of stomach acid, to solubilise the iron salts, into a form by which it can be absorbed by the intestines, if you are compensating in your bowel due to food intolerance, then the acid levels in you stomach, may not reach the PH required to break down the iron, so patently you will not absorb enough iron within your bowel, this could leave you with iron deficient anaemia, which is often found to be the case in food intolerants.

Before taking iron you should first consult a naturopathic Doctor, you should stop taking the iron if it upsets your system. I repeat if the iron makes you feel off or ill, or if there is a reaction to the iron then stop taking it.

I would advise you not to take any supplements, until you have consulted a Naturopathic Doctor, or someone qualified to assess your level of health. Self prescribing can be very harmful, and hinder recovery if the wrong types of medication are used.

DIGESTIVE TRACT REACTION

When we become intolerant to food we are in a catch 22 scenario, we are not extracting, absorbing and interacting vitamins and minerals properly, therefore we cannot create the correct gut flora to extract these vital vitamins and minerals properly, and thus catch 22 ensues, only persistence on the recovery programme will overcome these difficulties within the digestive tract and bloodstream.

I experimented whilst in the depths of my intolerance, taking all of the vitamins and minerals A, Bs, C, D, E, K, iron, zinc, selenium, folic acid, calcium etc, most of these seem to have little effect on my system, except for a couple of exceptions, the main one of these being vitamin E.

If you take vitamin E on its own, even 1- 400iu capsule of none wheat derived vitamin E, once every month, it has a very beneficial effect on your digestive system, especially in the early stages when you are extremely intolerant.

But if you take an excess of vitamin E in the early stages of recovery your digestive tract and detoxification system will not be able cope with it. This is probably due to your system trying to detoxify faster than the liver, kidneys, lymphatic and immune systems can cope, especially if you have Candida or yeast overgrowth. Vitamin E helps in detoxification, and many toxins can be released by the dying yeast overgrowth. Vitamin E is also an antioxidant, helpful in rebuilding tissue.

Another good element to take is zinc as this helps you to absorb what you eat more efficiently, and is a vital building block; Zinc can be taken from day one. There are a few types and occasionally people are affected by them, although this is very unlikely, so try one and if it does not have an adverse effect then it will be all right to take.

Later on in recovery you can take L-glutamine to help heal the digestive tract, don't take it in the early stages of recovery if you are extremely intolerant, your system won't cope with this, after saying this once you have recovered to the point where you can cope with the L-glutamine, your digestive system will be at the stage where it can heal itself, especially if you have begun to clean your system with the kidney cleanses and, gallbladder and liver flushes.

Vitamin C is also another element that will help to detoxify your system. Although if you are eating lots of fruit and especially vegetables, you shouldn't really need any supplement vitamin C. You could take some for the first month or so to kick-start recovery, the choice is yours.

If you are extremely intolerant do not take a multivitamin in the early stages of recovery, your system will react to it, as it cannot cope with the many elements and this will make you feel ill, there is also a possibility that the multi vitamins you choose could be bound with something that reacts with you, or the vitamin E in the multivitamins could be wheat derived.

Before taking any of these elements we need to take away the inflammation, and I found after much experimenting that this was best achieved in the main by diet alone, and eating lots of neutral foods, mainly rice, fruits, lean meats and vegetables, lightly cooked or steamed vegetables are even better, because they contain enzymes which help your digestive tract to break them down, you will find all this advice in the foods that can be eaten chapter, on pages 48-49, or the cut out wall chart on page 15.

There appears to be a very serious problem in the nutrient and vitamin absorption department, in that we are stuck in a controlled loop and are in the previously described catch 22 scenario, if you are extremely intolerant many nutrients begin to fall through the gut wall readily but in the wrong concentrations, this leaves you feeling tired and weak, as described in the what happens to the digestive tract chapter.

Although we begin to let many nutrients readily fall through the gut wall, some elements will be missing or malabsorbed, that is to say that our digestive tract has lost the ability to produce the correct gut environment to properly break down, extract convert, absorb, and interact these vitamin and mineral elements in the correct concentrations.

This is very serious, because without these elements, the digestive tract, and especially your liver, cannot function properly, and sustain the body's correct balance of nutrients, to synthesise efficiently, and repair itself.

So we have to try and break this loop scenario, but in the early stages of recovery if you are, or may be, extremely intolerant, taking multi vitamins will upset your system, this is why you should take away the intolerance foods first, as I have said before, by far the best way of stabilising your digestive tract in early recovery is by diet alone, other than taking the very few elements advised in the recovery programme, then judge how you feel after a month or so, if you are still experiencing symptoms such as stomach cramps and general stomach-ache then you may have Helicobacter Pylori, which you doctor can test for.

People often feel they should be taking something to aid in recovery, this is a mindset, through years of visits to the doctors and being prescribed something for even the mildest of ailments, when recovery would have taken place without them.

I say again, if you feel you should be taking a multivitamin do not take it in the early stages of recovery; let recovery get well under way first. Then and only then once recovery is well under way may you begin to tolerate a good multi vitamin without reaction, but by this stage of recovery you should not need a multi vitamin anyway.

There are only a few elements in a multi vitamin tablet that you may react with you, usually Stearic acid or wheat derived vitamin E, but in the early stages of recovery even this small amount will unhinge your system, and cause an adverse reaction.

I've made a point of "going on a bit" about this supplement issue because I find so many people reacting when first starting the recovery programme, and then I find that they are taking some multi vitamin supplements, and this is often the reason for their reaction.

There are only a few elements that I would advise you to take; and these are covered in the recovery programme.

PROBLEMS AT THE MOLECULAR LEVEL

I liken the complexity of the vitamin, mineral, and molecular interaction problem to building a pyramid with millions of playing cards, each card represents an interaction of two elements within the digestive tract, this pyramid is therefore made up of, and this is a guesstimate, sixteen million cards and thirty two million interactions, this being a multiple of the interactions based on the base vitamins, minerals and trace elements.

The complication occurs when you take away some of these cards, each of which represent an interaction, as the pyramid falls down you need to know which card or interaction fell next, and then next, and then next, to understand the consequence one reaction, or interaction, represented by each card will have on another, so as you can see the pyramid can fall down, in millions of different ways and combinations.

This is the problem when trying to solve intolerance from the molecular, there are so many paths of failure that if we know someone is short of one or other vitamin, or mineral, and we substitute it by giving them this element, or a drug, we can not be sure how it has affected the pyramid, if the crucial cards are not back in place, and exactly the right size, or we have imbalanced the pyramid, by putting in too much of the missing vitamins, or minerals, or drugs, and therefore the missing cards are too big, the pyramid will be imbalanced and will not stand up.

This is why many people who are given medication often say, my original condition or symptoms have gone away or subsided, but I now have two other side effects worse than the original condition, their pyramid is not in balance, their balance of vitamins minerals and nutrients is wrong.

Its far better to make sure your body has the correct tools to do the job, by making sure your digestive tract can function properly, by having a clean and efficient digestive tract you will extract nutrients, vitamins, and minerals efficiently, after all the body has spent millions of years learning how to interact all the vitamins, minerals and nutrients in the correct combination and order to keep the pyramid intact.

We may as human beings be intelligent, but I now believe it's about time we realised that the human body is far more intelligent than us, and when we try to redress an illness with medication, often all we are doing is tinkering at the edges, especially when it comes to common problems within the digestive tract, and many minor lifelong afflictions or conditions.

So unless all the organs responsible for the breakdown absorption and interaction of food, vitamins, and mineral elements work efficiently, then there is no way that the body can sustain and repair itself, and ward off minor illnesses and conditions, even everyday problems such as, The common cold, Flu, Thrush, Athletes foot, Candida Stomach ulcers, or even dare I say it, cancers etc.

Giving the body drugs to treat any given digestive condition, should only be advocated after you have recovered your digestive function, and you are absolutely confident and certain the body is working as efficiently as possible, but still cannot repair itself, without supplementing and aiding the bodily function, by the intervention of these drugs.

I feel sure that one day someone will be able to trace and map out the exact molecular interactions and elements involved in this complex problem, and thus unravel the chain reaction of gained food intolerance at the molecular level.

Although there is the possibility that the myriad of interactions in our digestive system may never let us fully unravel the complexities of food intolerance, and we may just have to accept that certain foods for many people cause food intolerance to develop, and allow the many related problems described in this book to develop.

ACKNOWLEDGMENT

"You are what you eat", well we may take this phrase for granted and eat and drink what we think is good for us and also what we prefere to eat and drink, but as I have learnt from the information in this book there is a lot of truth in those simple words.

Before I go any further I must say that I have worked alongside John Wrattall, the author of this book for fifteen years, and have seen him suffer poor health, which got so bad, he found he had to do something about it himself. Of course he at first whent along to his G.P. for help in his suffering as all of us would do. And after some time and frustration, he wasn't getting any better. So using a good old fashioned common sense approach with much time in researching, which is second nature to us as plant machinery engineers and is our profession, he has made himself better.

John being very sincere, helpfull and convincing I took an intrest in his progress and couldn't help. but see that I was suffering in a similar way and was feeding myself wrongly. Before this, like most of us, I thought I was on a good diet, but as symptoms creep up on us slowly over the years untill we start suffering from pain and discomfort, we don't do anything about it.

Untill now I didn't realise I was eating too much bread. which was bad for me, bread at breakfast time — as toast, for lunch in sandwiches and for tea and supper time. I ate bread with everything. I also thought it normal to feel tired after lunch and in the evenings and take tired a long while to 'come round' in a morning, in fact I was allways tiered, but without realising it I had learnt to cope with it so I could carry on with everyday life.

Knowing what I know now about diet from this book. I have cut down on bread drastically to eating the odd slice occasionally, plus eating more fresh fruit and veg. and try to avoid eating and drinking processed food, I now read the ingreedients on everything before deciding wether to eat it or not. As a result I feel more awake with more vitality, recover quickly from arduous physical excersise and above all feel younger. and hopefully will have less ill health as I grow older as a result. which I am sure by eating properly I will. After all us as humans are a product of nature designed to eat natural things, not processed food bombarded with chemicals wich overwork. and damage the human bodies already inbuilt ability to dispose of toxins.

I for one can do more to improve my diet and improve my ability to digest things properly, but I have made a start and have noticed some big improvements. This book explains everything in easy to understand terms with a natural cure for each symptom which must be benificial to most of us. What we eat is an important part of our lives which we have to take very seriously in order to live a healthy and fullfilling life I hope you all benifit as I have from reading this book.

Bernard Cookson.

HISTORY

It's only in our recent past that mankind, especially in the western world, has embarked unwittingly on a diet which is not altogether natural or compatible with our digestive systems.

The past 50 years in particular have seen a vast change in our everyday diet; much of our diet is processed and definitely incompatible with our digestive tract.

Mankind has only been eating large amounts of wheat, and dairy products for about the last 10,000 to 12,000 years.

If you took the length of time man has been evolving on this planet, and said it was 2,000,000 years, and then compressed it and represented it as a 24 hour day, then a quick calculation reveals that we have only eaten wheat, and dairy products, in larger quantities, for the last 7.2 minutes of the 24 hour day.

A more frightening statistic is revealed, if we look at our dramatic change in diet over the last 50 yrs or so, we have only been eating this intense barrage of fortified processed, preservative filled, refined, sugar laden, and unnatural diet for an infinitesimal amount of time, compared to the amount of time we have been evolving on this planet.

If you work out how long in the 24 hour day calculation this intense barrage has been eaten, it is equal to the last 0.36 of a second, in the twenty four hour day, this is positively, definitely, absolutely not long enough for our digestive tract to evolve and adapt to cope with our modern diet.

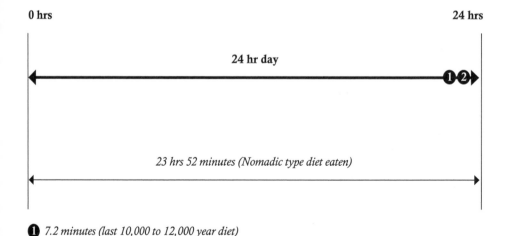

0 hrs   **24 hrs**

24 hr day

23 hrs 52 minutes (Nomadic type diet eaten)

❶ *7.2 minutes (last 10,000 to 12,000 year diet)*
❷ *0.36 seconds (last 50 years of diet)*

If we go back as little as ten to twelve thousand years, we find strong evidence that man was still in the main a hunter-gatherer.

This is to say that he wandered around to find his food and did not cultivate nurture or farm his food, he would have trapped or caught animals or fish, picked fruits or nuts from bushes and trees, grubbed vegetables and roots out of the ground, or took eggs from nests. In the case of wheat he would strip it from the stalk, and eat it in its rough state, and only when he found it growing wild, the only milk he would drink was probably his mother's milk as a baby.

THE WHEAT CONNECTION

Wheat twelve thousand years ago was an entirely different proposition, because it was wild wheat, and the grain would be much smaller, and very much less intense, and man would only eat small amounts stripped from the stalk in passing.

Modern varieties are much stronger and more intense, due to the domestication and selective cultivation of the grain throughout the last ten to twelve thousand years.

We have to remember that this was around the end of the last ice age, and mankind would find his natural environment changing rapidly, food in the natural environment would become less readily available and plentiful; therefore the hunter-gatherer, especially in more northern regions was forced to change his way of life.

He began to learn to cultivate and grow his own food, to substitute what he found growing in his natural environment.

This in turn would slowly change his diet, and he would become more reliant on cultivated products especially wheat, therefore his intake of these cultivated products would rise dramatically, over a short period of time.

This would not pose too much of a problem at first, because mankind would still not be eating it at every meal, and in an intensely fortified form, although his digestive tract would have to begin to adapt to his changing diet, and slightly change the way it functioned.

This the digestive tract can do, as long as it happens over a long period of time, tens of thousands of years, and not over one or two generations, or even 10 generations.

A very interesting fact in relation to wheat is that the Romans used to feed their slaves large quantities of wheat; this is because they had noticed that if you eat large quantities of wheat it makes you more lethargic and subdued. Therefore if they fed their slaves large quantities of wheat they would be more manageable.

The Romans may not have known the complexities of what was happening to the body, but they certainly observed the phenomena, and utilized the side effects of eating too much wheat for their own ends.

Now I have recovered, I eat very little wheat, but if I now eat a large quantity of wheat I can feel the effects, it definitely makes me slightly tired and lethargic, bearing out the observations that the Romans reported thousands of years ago.

THE DAIRY CONNECTION

Going back 1200 years and further into the past, our ancestors did not rear and domesticate cattle, and did not eat or drink dairy products, or certainly very rarely, although they would certainly have killed the occasional cow to eat its flesh.

There is no animal in nature that drinks the milk of another animal, so why should we be any different.

To eat the flesh of another animal is an entirely different thing, and historically much more natural.

When we are drinking mothers milk, we are ingesting milk with a different makeup to cows milk, mothers milk early in life is colonising our digestive tract with the bacteria and elements required, for proper breakdown and absorption of foods, and is also helping to set up our immune system, it is essential that a baby receives the first milk that mother produces, (colostrums), this is vital for initialising the immune system in an infant.

In our distant past mothers milk could have been the only milk that we ever ingested, and gave our systems the kick-start it needed in life.

MAN'S ENVIRONMENT

Things change very rapidly today.

There has been a compounding problem developing within our food environment for hundreds, if not thousands of years, but by far the most dramatic of these changes has developed over the last 50 years or so.

Our foods have changed enormously over the last two generations, and the digestive tract has not been able to keep up with these rapid changes.
It is an inescapable truth that our digestive tracts have not evolved or adapted, and gained the ability to break down our modern diet, in the little time that we have been eating it.

Before 10 to 12 thousand years ago, mankind would be much more likely to eat fruit, foods grubbed from the ground such as vegetables and roots, lean meats from the bird family, Eggs taken from nests, and oils and fats from catching and eating animals, or fish caught from shores or rivers.

All this would obviously be natural unprocessed food, and mankind would have been eating in this manner for hundreds of thousands or even two million years. Therefore his digestive tract had fine-tuned itself to this environment, and his digestive tract would be naturally able to break down, absorb, synthesise, and metabolise everything he ate efficiently.

Most of what he ate would be utilised by his body very efficiently, and very little toxic waste would be produced.

Obviously this would be far less stressful to the digestive tract than our modern diet.

One of the most detrimental appliances ever invented in relation to health, will prove in time to be the household fridge freezer. We can eat many readily available foods from the fridge or freezer, that even fifty years ago would not be available on tap.

We can eat meats and dairy products at will, and often indulge in these products at every mealtime-this is far from natural.

I am not saying don't use a fridge or freezer, but what I will say is be selective about what you eat from it and when, its not natural to slowly put oils and fats into your system in small amounts, and often at every meal.

If you go back thousands of years there were no fridges or freezers, you had to eat an animal you'd killed or a fish you'd caught there and then, or it would decay, therefore oils and fats would tend to be eaten at one or two meals, and probably on the same day.

The digestive tract then would be much more geared to this environment.

If we look at the gallbladder, this would be a larger organ then, and would be much more active. If you caught an animal you would have to eat as much of it as you could, simply because you had no means of keeping it for a prolonged period. Your digestive tract and particularly your liver and pancreas would have to produce large amounts of bile, enzymes and hormones to break down the oils and fats.

There are some distinct advantages in eating in this way, for instance this would have the effect of keeping the gallbladder clean, as it would in effect be very similar to what we are doing with the gallbladder and liver flush, in that it would force the liver to produce copious amounts of bile and store it in the gallbladder, so when large amount of oily, and fatty meat was eaten, the gallbladder would be primed and ready to squeeze all the bile out, this would help to wash out the gallbladder and keep the liver and bile ducts clean.

Meat, oil, and fat may not have been consumed for days after this, and the gallbladder would fill with bile, and the bile would become very concentrated, you would only have to break down the easily digested fruits, and grubbed up vegetables for a few days, with possibly the odd light meat, such as from a bird, the odd egg may also have been consumed.

This is how your body has developed for possibly two million years, and now over a few thousand years our diet has changed radically, and enormously, especially over the last 50 years, obviously our digestive system has adapted to some degree but it has not been able to keep up with the rapid change in more recent times.

You could almost say we are eating too well in this modern age. The body is not used to having all the vitamins and minerals all the time, this is why evolution has developed the body, and given it the ability to synthesise many of the foods we ingest, when it is short of one or other element or elements. (To synthesize is to change one and/or other elements into another element).

For instance, the body can synthesise sunlight and convert it into vitamin D, when the sun shines on you it converts 7-dehydrocholesterol into Vitamin D, and stores it in your liver, It can synthesise nutrients in your digestive tract and make vitamin B12, as long as your diet contains all the building blocks for these scenarios to take place.

Many of the modern so called diets, are vastly different to what would have been natural for mankind thousands of years ago.

For instance, to eat a vegetarian diet is not a natural diet, some oils and fats are necessary from an animal source, and it is definitely not natural to take supplements vitamins and minerals to maintain equilibrium in the digestive tract, and to maintain bodily function, cavemen did not have supplements, unless I'm missing something.

Ask yourself this question, if vitamin and mineral substitutes are necessary for modern man to stay healthy then how did mankind possibly survive until the twenty first century, without these vitamin and mineral substitutes.

We seem to assume these days that taking substitute vitamins and minerals is normal and an absolute requirement for health, survival and bodily function, if that is the case then how did mankind evolve through hundreds of thousands or even millions of years without them, don't you think it may have had something to do with his diet?

Are we really that naïve that we think we have to take substitute vitamins and minerals every day to stay healthy, look at your history?

I would agree that some trace elements are lacking due to modern agricultural methods, causing the depletion of certain trace elements in soils, but these trace elements are the only exception to the rule of vitamin and mineral substitutes, one such element is Zinc, very little or indeed none, is found in many tests conducted on modern agricultural land.

The best reason I can give you for adopting the advised recovery programme in this book, is that in effect, you will be eating what your body was in the past, naturally developed to ingest.

And if its going to be called a diet, then it should be called the stone age or caveman diet, because the foods I advise you to eat after full recovery, are basically what stone age or cavemen would have eaten.

All that I am asking you to eat are the foods that your body has evolved to eat, and digest, little wonder it begins to recover.

Although I have to say that the foods I advise you to eat in early recovery should initially be viewed as a recovery programme, and not a diet.

When you have fully recovered the best way to view this diet is to say to yourself, I'm not on a diet, I'm eating what mankind should be eating, it's the rest of the western world that's on a diet.

We should take great heed of our past history, and realize that evolution has not equipped our digestive tract to cope with our intense modern diet, of wheat, dairy and refined carbohydrate intake.

WATER CONSUMPTION

The problem with the modern diet is that it contains lots of dry matter, like pastry, pies, pizzas, bread etc, requiring us to take onboard more water than historically would be normal.

Historically, I mean beyond 12 thousand years ago, you would not drink lots of water every day, you would rely on getting most of your fluids from your diet, the last thing your ancestors wanted to do, would be to risk drinking contaminated water, from pools, still water etc, running or moving water would have been much safer for them to drink, and when they did drink, this is probably what they sought out.

It amuses me somewhat, when you see so many people walking around clutching a bottle of water in their hand, as if dehydration could strike at any moment, and their life depended on it. If you are fit and healthy your body tells you when it requires water, "you get thirsty".

Drinking too much water can be dangerous, as many athletes, especially marathon runners can testify, if they are sweating heavily they can deplete what are called electrolytes, and drinking just water does not replenish them, in extreme cases they may even collapse, and urgently require replacement electrolytes to regain normal function.

Your digestive tract recycles most of the water in it, and your kidneys only pass about 1 to 1 and 1/2% of the fluid in your body into your urine each day, so a fit and healthy body can extract most of the fluid it requires from the food you are eating, as long as you are eating lots of fluid laden fruit and vegetables.

THE KIDNEY CLEANSES

THE KIDNEYS AND KIDNEY STONES

The kidneys are a vital part of the detoxifying process, and therefore we need to make sure that they perform properly.

The kidneys are the blood filters of the body.

If you have extreme food intolerance and an open digestive tract as described previously in digestive compensation the emergency state, then your blood is going to be full of toxins and elements far in excess of what would be considered normal. This is going to overtax your kidneys, and filtration and detoxification will be impaired, leaving toxins piling up in your liver, kidneys and blood, this will make you feel ill and extremely tired.

That is why one of the first things to do after starting to eat the advised diet, is to clean out the kidneys. We need to recover the kidneys to help eradicate toxins, and ideally this should be done before embarking on any gallbladder flushes.

The first treatment that should be done in the early stages is the beetroot cleanse, the herbal cleanse is too severe in the early stages of recovery, and will overtax your ability to detoxify, so we will leave that for the later stages of recovery.

There are different types of kidney stones, some are formed from uric acid. Uric acid is formed from breaking down protein in the liver, there's lots of protein in the modern diet, especially wheat protein, hence uric acid type kidney stones.

These are also the more dangerous crystal type stones, these can cause severe damage to the kidneys and even kidney failure, crystals can even form in your joints and other tissues, and may give you the symptoms of gout, this is another reason why I make you eat less intense single protein (gluten) in your diet, whilst you are on the recovery programme.

There are other types of stones that can form such as amino acid stones, oxalic acid stones, and phosphate type stones, (calculi), these stones form as other failures in the digestive tract begin to develop, due to your intolerance to wheat, dairy and sugar, this begins to swamp the kidneys, and they can begin to amass these destructive elements.

All the previously mentioned type stones may be reduced or eradicated after some time on the diet and with the help of the second kidney cleanse using the herbs, as described on page 224.

You can also develop calcium type stones, formed through too much calcium in your system, and not enough magnesium to keep it in suspension, therefore the calcium is able to settle out in certain organs of the body, and in the case of the kidneys, calcium type stones may develop.

These are not as destructive and much more easily eradicated by the beetroot cleanse, as described in the kidney cleanse on page 223, again a good diet containing lots of fruit and especially vegetables will keep you free from calcium type stones in the future.

Beetroot contains lots of magnesium and helps to keep the calcium in suspension; this is why we use the beetroot juice in such a concentrated form in the kidney cleanse, it should help break down the calcium type kidney stones.

It is vital that the kidneys function properly, and therefore the kidney cleanses are a vital part of the recovery programme, and a must do, if full recovery is to take place.

WHEN DO YOU CLEANSE THE KIDNEYS?

I would advise you to do a beetroot type kidney cleanse, once in the early stages of recovery, usually after about one month, but before the end of the second month.
This first cleanse is before any gallbladder and liver flushes.

Then second beetroot type cleanse should be done after all the gallbladder and liver flushes required to flush the liver. This could be up to 16 months to 2 years, or even more if you are an extreme case.

The herbal type of cleanse should be done about a month after the second beetroot cleanse.

The herbal cleanse only needs to be done once, unless you have been extremely intolerant, then another herbal treatment at a later date is recommended.

So I repeat, do a beetroot type cleanse in the second month of recovery, and then after all of the gallbladder and liver flushes, do your second beetroot type cleanse, and then after about another month do the herbal type cleanse.

Whilst doing these cleanses try and keep off too many fats, preservatives, sugars or additives, try to eat only natural products.

This is all detailed in the recovery programme.

SYMPTOMS

The kidneys are responsible for the regulation of fluid, excretion of waste products, and the cleaning of the blood, so it's vital that we make sure that they function properly.

There are few obvious outward signs of kidney impairment, symptom are usually embroiled with the rest of the conditions in relation to food intolerance, but there are a few obvious symptoms.

• Gout or arthritic type symptoms (in depths of intolerance)

• Slight ache around lower ribcage when urinating.

• Slight aching in kidney area.

• Slight aching feeling swimming around rear midriff area of torso.

• Discharge of yellowish matter on penis in males, or vaginal thrush in women.

• Oily skin.

• Salty taste in mouth

• Slightly fluey sinuses

• Slight or general tiredness.

These kidney cleanses will help along with the other measures in this book to eradicate these symptoms, and dissolve any stones in the kidneys or ducting. They are so easy it would be silly not to do at least one course of kidney cleanses.

CAUSES

If you don't have enough magnesium in your system, your system cannot utilise all the calcium in your body.

This can result in surplus calcium forming calcium type stones in your kidneys.

If you eat lots of bread and dairy products, the dairy products contain lots of calcium, and the bread with its added calcium, are filling your system every day with excess calcium that the system cannot cope with, you will not have enough magnesium in your system to keep this excess amount of calcium in suspension, this can lead to calcium settling in the kidneys, and the development of calcium type kidney stones.

Many intolerants have usually built up calcium deposits on the inside of their bottom teeth for years, this is being secreted from the glands behind their bottom set of teeth, and every time they go to their dentist he will scrape these calcium deposits off, this is a graphic example of too much calcium in your system and not enough magnesium to keep it in suspension.

If you eat too much protein, as in wheat protein, and lots of bread every day, you will produce a lot of uric acid, nitrogen containing waste; this can be responsible for the formation of uric acid type kidney stones.

If you think back a number of years, can you remember if you had strong smelling, or strong acidic urine in your younger years? This is a good indication that your kidneys may have developed uric acid and related type stones, such as amino acid, oxalic acid, and phosphate type kidney stones.

If this is the case then the second herbal cleanse should help eradicate these, although it may have to be done twice, especially if you were extremely intolerant before starting the recovery programme.

This is not the sole cause of kidney stones, there are other more complex reasons for the formation of kidney stones, which are further covered in the, "what happens to the digestive tract" chapter. So it is absolutely vital that we clean out the kidneys, your system cannot function properly without having the ability to expel sodium, chlorine, calcium, potassium, phosphate, sulphate, urea, uric acid, creatinine, and amino acid, efficiently.

MY EXPERIENCE

I have no way of being certain whether I had kidney stones or not, but the treatment was certainly a vital tool in the recovery of my system, the slight pain experienced in my ureter area when urinating went away, and my urine was a dark yellow colour for about a week whilst taking the beetroot juice, and a brownish colour at the beginning of the herbal cleanse.

I also experienced some twinges in my lower abdomen whilst completing some of the cleanses, which I have to say stopped me in my tracks on two occasions whilst I was out walking, this only lasted for about two or three seconds, I am told this would be stones dissolving and moving out of the kidneys, or more likely have been, dissolving stones moving through the ureter. (Tubes from the kidneys to the bladder)

An excellent indication of dissolving stones is the presence of dark coloured urine, although this is not always the case.

Another extremely important and noticeable improvement, is in relation to the yeast overgrowth which can colonise the urinary tract, as well as your digestive tract, in women it will present as thrush, in men you may notice some accumulation of matter under the foreskin of the penis from time to time, but only if you are extremely intolerant, if you have these problems they will disappear completely after full recovery.

This second treatment definitely helps to clear up the condition in the urinary tract. This is a vital component in recovery, as the yeast overgrowth is one of the most stubborn conditions to eradicate, as detailed in the "yeast overgrowth or candida albicans" chapter page 164.

I have to say there was a definite and noticeable improvement in my well being after these kidney cleanses, and the yeast overgrowth receded to some degree.

Kidney stones can also affect many elements in the blood such as iron and salts, although you will only have this complication if you are in the more advanced stages of kidney problems, these cleanses helps to redress the balance and clean and stabilise your kidneys, and make them work more efficiently.

POSSIBLE REACTIONS

You may feel slightly tired whilst taking the beetroot juice; this is usually the only slight effect that is noticeable, other than maybe a slight ache in your kidney area, if you become really tired and weak then stop the beetroot cleanse and start again slowly.

The second cleanse, the herbal one, may make you feel stiff for about two to six days; this may occur after about a week into the treatment.

If you are killing off yeast overgrowth, which is basically a bacterium, and you are cleansing your kidneys, it may make you tired, because you have released many toxins into your system, and your system has to expel them, along with the elements released from the dissolving stones.
This may swamp your ability to detoxify for a few days.

So monitor the way you feel and back off with either of the two treatments for a few days if it makes you feel very tired, or you go very stiff. Make sure you drink plenty of water to dilute any toxins produced, by the cleansing action of the roots, in both the beetroot, and herbal cleanses.

THE BEETROOT CLEANSE

The remedy below is from a German doctor, and reportedly gives very good results; this treatment will help to eradicate calcium type kidney stones.

1 Wash clean six ordinary red beetroot but don't slice.

2 Boil the beetroot for one hour in six pints of water, slowly, so as not to boil the water away.

3 Bottle the water, place in the fridge to stop souring, if you cannot get fresh beetroot then buy canned beetroot and drink the water in the can.

4 Do not use any vinegar whilst drinking the beetroot water, as it will neutralise its effect.

5 Drink about half a cupfull or quarter of a mugfull three times a day, this dissolves the calcium type stones, they should just melt away, and not pass, its reported that hardly ever should a second treatment be necessary, you can use the same treatment to dissolve gravel in the bladder but it might require a longer treatment.

Important points for beetroot cleanse

• Do not take any vinegar, it will neutralise the effect

• Wash the beetroot but do not slice

• Try and keep off too many fats and additives

THE HERBAL CLEANSE

Do not attempt this cleanse in the early stages of recovery, the toxins it may release can swamp your ability to expel them, and may make you feel weak and tired.

Leave it until later on in recovery as detailed in "the recovery programme" chapter on page 80.

So, after the first and second beetroot cleanses, and any gallbladder and liver flushes, you can further, and vastly improve the condition or your kidneys by taking the following herbs over a period of 20-30 days.

These herbs are commonly used to aid the kidneys in recovery.

This cleanse is more related to cleaning the tissue of the kidneys, and is vital to recover the kidneys, and help to dissolve the uric acid, amino acid, phosphate, and oxalic acid build up in your kidneys, and should be done as the third treatment, after 16 months or so, and a month after the second beetroot cleanse, as I said before it is in "the recovery programme chapter" on page 80.

A second herbal cleanse may be necessary if you were extremely intolerant before beginning the recovery programme.

Below are the roots and herbs required for the treatment.
• 2 parts -BEARBERRY, arctostaphylos uva ursi

• 2 parts -HYDRANGEA ROOT, hydreanga officinale

• 1 part -GRAVEL ROOT, eupatorium purpureum

• 1 part -MARSHMALLOW ROOT, althea officianale

• 1 part -HORSETAIL, equisetum arvense

Method
• Take 100 Mg of each of the first two herbs, Bearberry and Hydreanga, and 50 Mg of the last three herbs, gravel root, Marshmallow root, and Horsetail, and mix them together.

• Keep them in a dry container.

• Before bedtime soak 4 or 5-heaped tablespoons of the mixture divided into three mugs of hot water, and leave overnight, the next morning bring to the boil, then let it simmer for 5 minutes then strain.

• Drink this mixture throughout the day; this does not need to be kept cool,

• Drink the juice between meals

• Do not add sweeteners.

• Drink plenty of water.

Important Points With Second Cleanse
- Do not sweeten

- Try to keep off too much fat

- Drink plenty of water

THE LEMON JUICE CLEANSE

I have included this lemon juice kidney cleanse in the book, but I would only advise you to try it after full recovery, the problem with this cleanse is the three days where you eat no food at all, those of us who are extremely food intolerant cannot cope with three days without food whilst in recovery, it will leave you exhausted, and you will not cope with the levels of lemon juice you are required to drink, without causing upset in your digestive tract.

You will be better doing this cleanse if you can have three or four days off work, this will give you a much better chance of completing the cleanse successfully.

A naturopathic doctor informed me of this cleanse, she has tried it on clients and it worked, these clients had been scanned and told they had kidney stones, after taking the lemon juice for three days they were scanned again, and told that their kidney stones had gone.

I would not advise you to do this cleanse on your own, you really need to do it under the supervision of a naturopathic doctor.

This lemon juice cleanse is very simple, but not easy, you will be craving food after the first day, and desperate for food after the second.

Lemon Juice cleanse pointers
- Do not eat excessive amounts of food the day before you start this cleanse.

- Do not eat any food for the three days of the treatment.

- On each of the three days put 500 ML of lemon juice into 2 litres of water, and drink through out the day.

- On the fourth day you can resume eating normally.

Warning
Please consult a naturopathic doctor before attempting this cleanse.

CONCLUSION AND THE FUTURE

You can buy beetroot in their own juice from supermarkets, usually shrink wrapped, it is advisable to have these whenever you have a salad, this should be enough to maintain freedom from calciate type kidney stones in the future, as long as a good diet is also adopted.

A good diet should also prevent you from forming the harmful elements related to the herbal cleanse, such as the uric acid, amino acid, phosphate, and oxalic type kidney stones.

These cleanses are well worth doing, all these cleanses are painless, and are a "must do" to aid in the recovery process.

If your kidneys don't function properly you will never recover 100%.

THE GALL BLADDER AND LIVER FLUSH

Please read this entire chapter and fully understand it, to familiarise yourself with the possible scenarios involved, then you will understand the flush fully, and what to expect when flushing.

The flush is also referred to as a gallbladder and liver cleanse on many internet sites.

WHEN NOT TO FLUSH

I would advise you not to attempt a flush, if you are experiencing any of the following.

- If you are very constipated (LESS THAN ONE BOWEL MOVEMENT EVERY THREE DAYS AND DIFFICULTY PASSING STOOLS) then you are advised to see a Naturopathic Doctor, to regain some normality of bowel movement before attempting a flush.

- Flu

- The common cold.

- Before starting the diet.

- Being treated for, or are on medication for liver problems.

- Being treated for or are on medication for kidney problems.

- Have had hepatitis B, within the last four years.

- Have known heart problems.

- Within twelve months of having your gallbladder removed.

- If you are a Diabetic, you may do the flushes, but do not drink the apple juice, take malic acid for the before the flush instead. (I would advise you to consult a Naturopathic Doctor)

- If you are under 15 years old.

- If you have in your past, had any blockage in your bowel.

- If you have had a bowel resection within the last twelve months.

WHEN SHOULD YOU FLUSH?

This should only be done after 2 to 3 MONTHS on the diet.

The only exception to this rule, is if you have been close to this diet for some time before starting this recovery programme, in which case you may begin cleansing much earlier, after 4 to eight weeks on the diet.

Why after two to three months on the diet?

Because we need to stabilize your digestive tract with the diet, and settle any inflammation before we begin the flushes.

You will also loose any water retention, and your immune system will recover to some degree, and your lymphatic system will also recover to some degree.

This stabilisation and partial recovery of your digestive and detoxification system is vital before beginning to flush.

This will also teach you the importance of the diet, if you step off the diet you will very quickly realize the consequences, you will experience tiredness, stomach ache, bloating, aching joints and other recurring symptoms.

This diet will have to be adopted until all the flushes necessary have been completed.

You should leave 5 to 6 weeks between flushes, THE ONLY EXCEPTION TO THIS 5 TO 6 WEEK RULE, is if you do not get all the gallstones out, that were in a position to be flushed out, then the ones still in your ducting will still be blocking your ducts, and leave you blocked up immediately after a flush.

You will know if this situation occurs, because you will feel slightly full after food, your stools may go loose and light coloured, you will feel lethargic, you may experience other gallstone symptoms (listed below) again within two to three days,

Once you have done a few flushes you will learn what to expect after a flush, and will instinctively know if you have not flushed out all the gallstones,that were able to be flushed out.

If the main bile ducting is clear after a flush, which it usually is, it can take days or even weeks for more stones to drift down from the minor ducting in your liver, and impede your main bile duct again, where they will then be in a position to be flushed out, this is why we leave 5 to 6 weeks between flushes.

The following gives an exhaustive list of possible symptoms.

POSSIBLE SYMPTOMS OF GALLSTONES

• Aching and stiffness in shoulders, more in the right one. (in advanced cases)

• Bloated stomach.

• Chest pains, pains around chest area, (in advanced cases) (If you have a tight chest like someone is sat on it, and this is accompanied by pain in and under your left arm, then please consult your family doctor immediately)

• Constipation (if partially blocked)

• Hypoglycaemia (low blood sugar, in advanced cases, pre diabetic state)

• Dry bottom lip.

• Flatulence

• General tiredness and lethargy.

• Itching all over, not all the time but on regular occasions.

• Jaundice. (yellowy appearance, in advanced cases)

• Light coloured stools, or switching between light then dark stools, (very good indication of clogged liver)

• Lines or ridges running the length of your fingernails.

• Lost sense of thirst (in extreme cases)

• Lower back ache.

• Loose bowels (if very blocked)

• Mouth ulcers, often inside bottom lip, (in advanced cases)

• Oily skin, especially around bridge of nose, and forehead.

• Slight pain or dull ache under lower right hand ribcage, (often associated with I.B.S)

• Tan easily in sun.

• Tiredness

• General wind.

- Pain in back between shoulder blades, more under your right shoulder blade, especially in the morning after sleep, and for a time after rising, (these symptoms are more pronounced in the extremely advanced cases, many flushes will be required)

- Red hue in whites of eyes.

- Pain under your front lower right rib cage, and in extreme cases possibly running around your right hand side and even as far as under your right shoulder blade.

- Slight nausea or pain, especially after eating oily or fatty foods.

- Slightly blocked sinuses, or a slight cold all the time.

- Splitting and dryness of the bottom lip.

- Dry skin at left, and right edges of mouth.

- Yeast overgrowth, (yellowish white on back of tongue, 99% of people with gallstones have yeast overgrowth, Candida)

If you don't have any of these symptoms, then you may not have gallstones. Or should I say if you have gallstones they are not yet giving you any symptoms.

If you have been scanned and gallstones are found, then it's either a flush, or the alternative is surgery. I know which I would prefer.

A scan may, but does not always detect gallstones, and will definitely not show up a clogged liver, this is yet another reason for a flush.

Surgery involves removing the entire gallbladder, or removing the stones from it with keyhole surgery, and then the gallbladder itself.

The problem with this approach is it does not clean the liver of chaff and sludge, or retained gallstones in the liver or ducting, or the crystals, which are the early formation of gallstones.

Many people have their gallbladder taken away, and continue to have digestive problems, this is because the liver and ducting is still coagulated and partially blocked, leaving them with an impaired free flow of bile from the liver, and throughout the entire bile duct.

These people require their liver cleaning out, before they will regain the ability to break down the intolerance foods again, wheat and dairy products etc.

If you have had your gallbladder removed, then I would advise you not to embark on a flush until twelve months or so after your operation, this is to make sure you have healed properly first.

If you are reading this book, and you know anyone who has had their gallbladder removed, and are still experiencing symptoms, such as bloating, gaseousness, I.B.S symptoms, then have a word with them, it is more than likely that their liver is still clogged, and a series of flushes is recommended, but remember they must only commence with the flushes, twelve months after any gallbladder operation, to make sure they are healed properly, they must also adopt the diet in this book to stabilise their digestive tract before cleansing.

I have had people who have been scanned for gallstones and told, "you definitely do not have gallstones" However after monitoring their symptoms, I was convinced they had gallstones, and subsequently after some persuasion they have done a gallbladder and liver flush and flushed out hundreds of gallstones, and had to do eight or ten flushes to clean the liver properly.

Only then have their symptoms receded, and their breakdown and absorption pattern improved dramatically.

If you have yeast overgrowth, (candida) then a gallbladder and liver flush is essential, this is a good indication that you may have gallstones, or at least a clogged liver.

Some people have gallstones and never experience any outward symptoms or pain at all, the first sign that you may have a clogged liver is the increasing awareness that some foods affect you if you eat them, usually wheat or dairy products, so if you are beginning to be affected by certain foods, then a gallbladder and liver flush is essential.

This flush is vital to repair your digestive system, and to make sure there are no hidden stones or chaff in your liver or ducting, impairing bile production and consequently breakdown and absorption of foods.

A minimum of three flushes is recommended, or as many as required to clean the liver of gallstones and chaff, if you are extremely intolerant you may need as many as twenty flushes, although this is unusual, I have only had five people who have had to complete in excess of twenty flushes to clean their liver.

I had to complete twenty six flushes before my liver was clean, and I regained a free flow of bile again

SYMPTOMS OF BECOMING BLOCKED BETWEEN FLUSHES

If you have hundreds, or possibly thousands of gallstones, your common bile duct will slowly become blocked again after each flush, or until you have completely flushed out all the stones and chaff.

Some of the obvious symptoms will probably include!

• Slight pain just under your ribcage, and slightly to the right of centre.

• If you become very blocked you may experience slight aching, right across your stomach area, and the discomfort may be more apparent after food.

• Flatulence.

• Oily on bridge of nose and forehead.

• The whites of your eyes may be pink when first rising in the morning, and slightly pink throughout the day.

• You may have a slightly tanned appearance in your face.

• If you feel a slight pain under your right lower shoulder blade, this is an indication that you still have some stones or chaff, and you will definitely require another flush.

Occasionally you may begin to experience stomach ache and symptoms within two to three days of completing a flush, this is usually because many stones have rapidly moved down and partially blocked your bile ducting again, if you experience symptoms very quickly after a flush, you will have to complete another flush after as little as a week, this flush will be deemed an emergency flush.

If this scenario presents itself you will not need to drink apple juice for five days before the flush, you can just complete the flush as if you are doing the final day of the flush, the sixth day, by having an early lunch, taking the Epsom salts and the olive oil etc, as detailed in the last day of the flush. This is the only time you are allowed to complete a flush within five weeks of a preceding flush, and should not be adopted on a regular basis.

MY EXPERIENCE

I did not realise I had the symptoms of gallstones until I took all the intolerance foods away. The bloating and related aches and pains whilst in the depths of intolerance were masking the gallstone symptoms, after 12 to 14 months the bloating and many other symptoms as listed on pages 18 to 21 had gone, and the gallstone symptoms were only mild, and were the only symptoms I was left with.

After about 12 to 14 months I realised that I was not breaking down foods properly, and thought it could be a gall bladder problem, as I discussed in the symptoms chapter.

So I approached my doctor to consider a gall bladder scan, but after some discussion he thought it unlikely I would have gallstones, and did not consider a scan necessary.
But after I had insisted on a scan he relented and I had an ultrasound scan.

To my amazement I was told I did not have gallstones, but was told my gallbladder appeared a little odd, in that it was not smooth on the outside as expected, but looked lumpy.

But I was still convinced that I had gallstones, I thought to myself I will have to find another way, and so I spent a month or so trying to find an alternative cure for gallstones.
After trying some and dismissing many treatments as non-starters, my sister Janet came across one that after some studying I thought might just work.

So, I tried this gall bladder flush, and to my amazement passed over 2400 stones, yes 2400, but I had to do 26 flushes, 120 were as large as a large pea, about 1200 as large as a pin head, there were hundreds of others too soft to collect, and in the early flushes some were made of grit, small in size and black, in the latter flushes I passed lots and lots of chaff.

If you collected all these stones and chaff they would have filled a half pint glass, little wonder my liver did not function properly, leaving me unable to break down food properly.

My doctor did me a favour when he eventually sent me for a scan, and no gallstones were found, if they had found them on the scan I would probably have had my gallbladder taken out.

It was only after I had cleaned my gallbladder and liver out, that I began to develop the theories discussed in this book, and begin to unravel some the complexities of the digestive tract in relation to the liver and gallstones.

It was only after working out this problem that it began to dawn on me that most people with I.B.S, , M.E (yuppie flu) and many other digestive tract problems, such as diverticulitis, crohns disease, ulcerative colitis, duodenal and peptic ulcers, probably all have the same causal factor, which is poor diet, leading to clogging of the liver, and consequentially the aforementioned digestive conditions.

I have now proven this theory with the many people who have had these conditions, adopted the recovery programme, completed the flushes in this book, and have subsequently fully recovered.

MINOR PROBLEMS WHEN FLUSHING

You may find that whilst you are holding your leg up towards your chin, your foot and lower leg go numb, so you may need to straighten your leg every 5 minutes or so, just for a minute or two to get the circulation going again, resume the position again afterwards and the oil will continue to drain from the stomach.

You may experience stomach-ache and feel nauseas in the night whilst doing a flush, and it may possibly make you vomit, although this is very unusual.

The main reason why you may feel ill in the night, is due to the fact that you have eaten some food too close to the run up to the flush, this will give you stomach ache and may on rare occasions even make you vomit, so its important not to eat anything after a light early lunch on the day of the flush.

The other reason why you may feel nauseas, is because you have drunk too much olive oil, you only need the amount recommended in the details of the flush.

On the run up to the flush whilst drinking the apple juice, you may experience feeling a little off for a day or two, this is quite normal.

If the apple juice gives you a pain in your lower abdomen, then eat 4 apples a day instead of the apple juice, and take the apple juice on the fifth day only, and then only half a litre.

On the second and subsequent flushes, you should not need to drink anywhere near as much apple juice, about half to one litre a day is enough.

Stay relatively fat free for three days after the flush, especially the first three flushes, you may have flushed out lots of gallstones, these are in your digestive tract, they are made up mainly of cholesterol, and some of it will be absorbed by your system.

This excess cholesterol may give you a tight chest for a day or two, after the stones are flushed out, so we don't want to add to it by eating anything fatty or oily. Although its only if you have been extremely intolerant that you may experience a tight chest.

It may take a few days for your system to stabilise again, but no discomfort will be felt, you may just feel a little off for a day or so.

THE FLUSH

I now include the flush in the recovery programme, just to make sure that if you have gallstones you get them out, it is essential that you have a free flow of bile from the liver down and through the common bile duct.

Hundreds of thousands of people have done this without resorting to major surgery; even keyhole surgery is not always successful because they are not getting the chaff and residual gallstones out of the liver or ducting, often surgery will take the pain away but still leave you with many symptoms.

An impaired liver also interferes with the production and free flow of enzymes from the pancreas.

A fully functioning liver is vital for good health, and as I've said before you must do at least three flushes, it can in rare cases take three flushes to loosen the stones, and begin to release them, if you do get gallstones out then you must keep doing flushes until you have got them all out, you must then continue flushing until you get all the chaff out.

Usually you will pass the green coloured stones at first and they will slowly become less green and more tan coloured as more flushes are completed.
On the first flush you may flush out some cream or tan coloured stones, although this is not the norm, this would indicate that you probably only have a few gallstones and not many flushes will be required.

When doing the latter flushes you will begin to flush out the chaff, this is more important than the stones and you must flush until you get out all the chaff.
I repeat you must keep cleansing until the liver is clear of stones, and more importantly chaff.

If after the flush you do pass many gallstones and or chaff, the stones will be green, and the chaff is tan coloured, as in the examples at the end of this chapter, they are mainly made up of cholesterol.

You may find as I did that you get many stones out after the first flush. However you will need to do the minimum of three, possibly up to ten or even twenty if you are extremely clogged up, keep flushing at five to six week intervals until you stop passing stones and have cleaned out all the chaff, then you know you've got everything out.

A couple of months or even six months after you have done what you thought was your last flush, you may get the symptoms back again. This is because some stubborn gallstones and mainly chaff that was stuck high in your liver, have moved down into your gallbladder, and bile ducts, and blocked them again, this will require another flush, and will probably be the last flush you need.

Although I would recommend you do a flush on a regular basis, usually once or twice a year.

You may not find any gallstones on the first flush, but check and be sure; you may have passed some chaff or cream coloured stones, in which case you will have to keep cleansing, until all the chaff has been removed.

As I've said before sometimes it can take up to three flushes to loosen the gallstones, and before you begin to pass them, and get them on the move. This is the reason why I cannot over emphasise the importance of doing at least three flushes, and then keep doing flushes until no more gallstones are passed.

WHAT IS THE APPLE JUICE DOING?

You will drink apple juice, or eat apples for five days on the run up to the flush, the reasons why we drink apple juice are, firstly, to try and break down the cholesterol coagulation between the stones, and loosen them before we flush, and secondly to give the liver a store of glycogen in readiness for the flush.

The malic acid in the apple juice, latches onto the cholesterol coagulation between the stones, and release them.

We are also going to give the liver a good store of glucose to work with when we flush, because the apple juice also contains sugars, these scenarios plus the fat free diet means that the liver is virtually shut down, it's only ticking over for the five days on the run up to the flush, and therefore is primed and waiting to be switched on by the olive oil.

WHAT ARE THE EPSOM SALTS DOING?

Next you will drink the Epsom salts, this will dilate and open the common bile duct, giving any bile and/or gallstones a free unrestricted passage throughout the entire bile duct.

The salts will also give you very loose bowels, and expel any food remaining in your digestive tract, when the gallstones are flushed out of your liver they will also have a free passage and will be washed through your entire digestive tract.

WHAT IS THE OLIVE OIL DOING?

Finally you will drink the olive oil and lemon juice, or grapefruit juice mixture, when your liver detects this oil in your duodenum, it will be triggered and will release copious amounts of bile which will flood down the already open bile ducts, washing any gallstones or chaff from your gallbladder and lower liver, into your digestive tract.

WHY YOU NEED TO LIE ON RIGHT AND LEFT SIDE'S AND PULL YOUR KNEE UP?

The reason why you must go to bed immediately after drinking the olive oil, and then firstly lie on your right hand side, with your right knee pulled up towards your chin, is to distort the valve in the bottom of your stomach, (pyloric valve) and thus encourage the olive oil and grapefruit mixture to pass into your duodenum, the common bile duct from your live flows into your duodenum, the oil needs to be in your duodenum for your liver to be triggered, when the oil is detected by cells in your duodenum they release hormones which trigger your liver and gallbladder to release copious amounts of bile.

After lying on your right side for twenty minutes you will then turn onto your left side, and pull your left leg up towards your chin for twenty minutes, this will have the effect of pulling the common bile duct straight, giving a free passage for any gallstones or chaff, this will also allow gravity to help in draining the liver of gallstones and/or chaff.

You may now sleep normally.

NB.
After the first three flushes it is not necessary to pull you knees up towards to your chin.

THE GALLBLADDER AND LIVER FLUSH (VERY IMPORTANT)

THE FIRST 5 DAYS

1 On the first flush drink 1 litres of apple juice daily for 5 days prior to the flush (normal juice from shops, eat normally but fat free)

2 On subsequent flushes half to one litre of apple juice daily is sufficiennt.

3 If apple juice affects you eat four apples a day instead of drinking the apple juice.

4 If you are diabetic eat one apple a day instead of the apple juice, and take malic acid tablets, (as directed on the malic acid container)

5 Stay on the diet but eat as fat free as possible for these 5 days.

THE DAY OF THE FLUSH, 6TH DAY

On the sixth day, do not eat anything after an early light 11.30 lunch

1 Have a light early lunch 11 to 11.30 Am, nothing after lunch, and no evening meal, you may drink water.

2 At 8 pm take 3 level teaspoons of epsom salt, dissolved in a mug of warm water, (if you don't like the taste of them and cannot drink the epsom salts in a full mug of water, then dissolve them in a small amount of warm water and drink them, and then drink a mug of warm water after, or try drinking them using a straw, or holding your nose, this bye passes most of your taste buds)

3 At 9 pm take another 3 level teaspoons of epsom salt. (Use any of the previous methods to get them down)

4 At 10 pm, mix 80-120 ml or a quarter to a third of a mug of olive oil, with the juice from 2 freshly squeezed lemons, or 150 ml of lemon juice from shops, and then drink it all down. Extreme food intolerants may react to lemon juice in early recovery, so alternatively you could use grapefruit juice, as long as you are not on medication which will react with grapefruit.

5 Immedietly upon finishing the olive oil, and lemon juice, or grapefruit juice, go to bed.

6 Then, lie on your right side, with your right knee drawn up towards your chin for twenty minutes.

7 Then, lie on your left side with your left knee drawn up towards your chin for twenty minutes.

8 And now go to sleep as normal.

THE DAY AFTER THE FLUSH

1 Next morning the stones will pass, there may be grit or gallstones cream or green in colour and soft as putty, varying in size from grains of sand to some as large as your thumb nail, you will not feel a thing but will be amased with the results.

2 Stay fat free for three days after flush

3 On the fifth day after each flush take 400iu of Vitamin E

Important notes

1 For five days prior to flush eat as fat free as possible.

2 No food after 11.30am on day of flush.

3 Go to bed immediately after taking the oil and lemon juice, and lie on right side with right leg   drawn up to your chin, and then left side with left leg drawn up to your chin.

4 Its vital that you whisk your stools in the toilet pan, then let it settle, and identify any floating stones, then you know what to look for on subsequent flushes, and know when you have flushed out all the stones and chaff.

5 Stay fat free for 3 days after the first couple of flushes, it's not so critical to stay fat free after the later flushes.

6 If you are a diabetic do not drink the apple juice, eat one apple a day instead, and take malic acid.

7 Five days after each flush take 400 iu of Vitamin E.

8 At the risk of becoming boring i shall emphasise yet again you must do at least 3 of these flushes. Some people don't begin to flush out any stones until the third flush. The first two flushes are loosening the stones. However most people pass stones on the first flush.

RETRIEVING THE STONES AND CHAFF

On the first flush, and so that you learn to recognise gallstones, I would recommend you to whisk your stools in the toilet pan and identify any stones present.

Use a food whisk or something similar, (no not an electrical one, a hand held one) the cholesterol type stones will float on the water, and be recognisably green or tan in colour.
Any tan coloured chaff will also float.

You usually find that you pass some more stones the first time you pass a stool again, this may be the day after the flush, or may even be two or three days after doing a flush, so it is a good idea to whisk your stools for the first day or two after a flush, and see if there are any more stones, or chaff floating in the toilet pan.

WHAT ARE YOU LOOKING FOR?

• Green coloured, pin head, pea, fingernail or thumbnail sized stones.

• Cream coloured stones, usually these are about 1-2 MM across but can be up to the size of your small fingernail, these are often referred to as soap stones.

• Small black stones, these are very hard and rough about 1-2 MM in size.

• Gravel, which is similar in appearance to sand.

• Chaff on the last flushes required, this will be very small and green the same colour as the gallstones, or it will be a tan colour and very small, about 1-2mm across, often on the last flushes you may find it difficult to ascertain what is chaff.

• Chaff will float and can sometimes appear as a fatty floating scum or mush, or the previously mentioned very small green or tan coloured stones, or even very small cream coloured soap stones, sometimes you find chaff in the form of small slivers, like rolled up tomato skins or small ears of corn.

EXAMPLES OF STONES AND CHAFF

• The green ones are the ones you will pass in the early flushes. If they are very old gallstones they will be more polished and more uniform in shape, and a very dark green colour.

• The later ones are rougher on the surface, lighter green, and you may find they have some cyan and yellow colour in them after some flushes.

• The cream coloured ones are waxy and soft, and are often referred to as soap stones, these are also made of cholesterol.

• The varying colours of these gallstones can be seen on the bar chart on the rear cover of this book.

SHAPE OF GALLSTONES

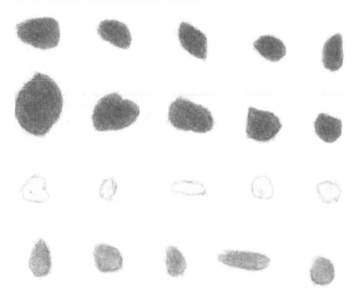

The tan coloured ones will indicate that you are nearly there, very small tan and light green stones are usually mixed in with the chaff on later flushes, and the last of the stones to be flushed out, this will then be followed by the mushy mud like chaff and/or chaff that looks like ears of corn, the liver should then be clean and able to recover fully over the period of a few months.

Again the varying colours of these can be found on the back cover of this book.

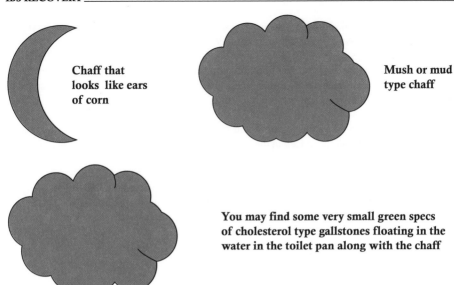

Chaff that looks like ears of corn

Mush or mud type chaff

You may find some very small green specs of cholesterol type gallstones floating in the water in the toilet pan along with the chaff

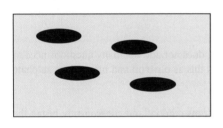

You may find some sand or gravel type stones on the first flush. This can vary in colour from a dark sandy colour to a light sand colour, or even a grey colour. There may also be some hard black stones, about a 1/16th of an inch across.

WHAT CAN YOU EXPECT, AND FIND AFTER A FLUSH?

It is unusual but on your first flush you may find you flush out lots of the cream coloured stones, these will be about the size of a pea and very soft, these are the early formation of gallstones.

If you flush lots of these out, it is a good sign that you don't have too many gallstones, and will probably get away with 3 or 4 flushes

Also on the first flush you may find some of the small black stones. The small black ones are made up of a very hard grit like material, you will also probably pass some gravel, this is like sand, and can vary in colour between grey and tan or the colour of dark sand.

Normally on the first and subsequent flushes you will find green coloured stones, about the size of a pea or up to the size your fingernails or thumbnail.

The green stones are the ones you will find until you begin to pass chaff, which could be after as many as ten or in the extreme twenty flushes, these green stones may have some electric blue, cyan, and yellow colour hidden in the recesses in the stones.

I repeat yet again keep doing flushes, until you find that you start passing and flush out all the chaff, this is a light tan colour, and about the size of large pinheads, some may be in small slivers or even mush.

Its imperative that you get all the chaff out, this is more important than the gallstones. A good indication of having cleaned out the stones and or chaff from your main ducts, is your stools will go darker in colour, until after a few days or weeks when you may begin to block again as more stones pass into your main bile duct, in which case another flush will be required.

ARE THEY GALLSTONES

There is some controversy about gallstone, when doctors see the gallstones which patients take for them to have a look at, "they all say yes those look like gallstones", but without having them analysed they often state that it is only congealed olive oil and Epsom salts creating stones that are similar in form to gallstones.

This anomaly requires further investigation, something does not add up, many questions need to be answered before the medical profession just dismiss this as olive oil and magnesium sulphate congealing in the digestive tract.

One patient I was working with fulfilled all the symptoms criteria, and consequently began the recovery programme detailed in this book, he completed one liver and gallbladder flush, and green stones were observed in his stools the day after the flush, which is normal after a flush.

About six weeks later he suddenly developed severe stomach ache and vomiting after eating food, the pain was so debilitating and intense he went to A and E, where he was observed for a day and discharged with a suspected stomach bug.

The next day he began eating again and the same symptoms recurred, he returned to A and E, doubled up in agony and vomiting, I suspected this could be a rolling intussusception, he was kept in hospital for five days, no scans or intervention were carried out.

He was so afraid of recurring symptoms that he ate no food for five days, and was then discharged, he then began eating small amounts of food again, and initially had some stomach discomfort, but not recurring severe pain.

If this had been an intussusception then it was idiopathic.

About a week after being discharged from hospital he began to pass green stones in his stools, no gallbladder and liver flushes were undertaken, this continued for about two weeks every time he passed a stool, after he stopped passing these stones he reported feeling much better with more energy, and can now eat some wheat and dairy with no reaction.

This is an extremely interesting case, the green stones could not have been a combination of olive oil and magnesium sulphate, so what were they?, was it the liver releasing a substance of some kind, and congealing in the digestive tract, was it because he did not eat anything for five days, changing the environment within his digestive tract, we will probably never know.

It was only after this event that he reported feeling much better, with more energy, and even climbed England's highest peak (Scafell pike) a few weeks later.

The following questions require answering, before an absolute answer can be ascertained with regard to gallbladder and liver flushes.

• Why, do patients often not pass gallstones until they have completed two or three flushes.

• Why, once the liver is clean do patients not create any more gallstones after doing a flush.

• Why, after each flush do patients report feeling progressively better.

• Why, do some patients only require 5 flushes, and can then eat anything without symptoms, but extreme food intolerants may require 40 flushes.

• Why, do patients not progress in their recovery if they do not complete any liver flushes.

• Why, do patients react differently to each flush,

• Why, do you only begin to flush out chaff (sludge) in the latter flushes, and often in mid recovery cream coloured or tan coloured stones are only flushed out.

• Why, does stomach bloating only begin to diminish as each flush is completed and recovery is under way.

• Why, don't other symptoms such as, photo sensitivity, tinea pedis, IBS, celiac disease (late onset), aching joints (especially synovial), myalgia, neuralgia, candida albicans, skin palpitations, fluid retention, anxiety, anaemia, constant fatigue, poor memory, headaches, back ache usually at L 4,5, and many more symptoms not subside if no gallbladder and liver flushes are completed.

Why, don't serious conditions such as diverticulitis, ulcerative colitis, ulcers (duodenal or gastric) Crohns, colonitis, not improve dramatically until some gallbladder and liver flushes have been completed. The dietary changes improve these conditions dramatically, but change to the point of recovery does not take place unless flushes are undertaken.

All these questions need to be addressed by the medical profession, and not just dismissed as another alternative medicine that is hogwash, it is about time that common sense began to prevail, patently something is happening when flushes are undertaken, and it is not at a psychiatric problem or abstinence from intolerant foods resting the digestive tract, which is often suggested as being the explanation.

There is a definite and observable change in the patient's well being if this recovery plan is undertaken.

The prognosis would be very poor if the flushes were not embarked upon.

I have to say that the vast majority of patients whom I see, say to me, that they, the medical profession that is, are not listening to me, they dismiss my problems and make me feel like a hypochondriac, their attitude is awful, but I have to say that the medical professions attitude is often born out of frustration because they do not have the answers to digestive issues where no measurable definable datum point can be established.

Therefore treatment is often palliative and therefore no improvement or recovery is observed.

Why don't the medical profession say, look I am sorry but we don't seem to have an answer to your problem, instead of being aloof and condescending to their patients and not seeming to sympathise with their plight.

CONCLUSION

You will find a vast improvement in your condition very rapidly once you have cleaned your liver properly.

I now definitely break down foods much efficiently, and more importantly absorb foods much better, and therefore have more energy and vitality.

So, a flush is well worth doing and is necessary to recover the ability of your digestive tract to break down, extract, and absorb foods much more effectively.
Its well worth the slight discomfort you may experience.

Some people have no discomfort at all and just pass the stones feeling no nausea at all, the lucky devils.

Once you are fully recovered it may be advisable to undertake a flush at regular intervals, say once or twice a year.

I would even go so far as to say that everyone should do a gall bladder flush every year, or even twice a year, especially with the modern western diet, of fast and processed foods, although the diet you are finally on after reading this book, should not be viewed as a diet, it is what you should be eating, and have evolved and adapted to eat, it's the rest of the western world that is on a diet.

Oh and bye the way if you get stones out its well worth collecting the large ones in a sealed glass jar, it makes quite a good party piece to show people your stones, but please not whilst the buffets on!

THE IN DEPTH MEDICAL EXPLANATIONS

You may be interested in reading about the digestive tract in more detail, so in this chapter I will explain in more depth, and with some medical terminology, some of the understanding, observed reactions and conclusions drawn from all my experimenting on myself and others, this will lead me to make some quite radical statements in this chapter, and bring into question some of the conventional understanding of how the digestive tract functions.

Digestive function is not an exact science but I now know that diet must be changed when digestive function is impaired, this will stabilise the situation, and then recovery of the digestive tract can be initiated, using gallbladder and liver flushes and kidney cleanses.

CONVENTIONAL UNDERSTANDING

The following few pages are just to recap on the digestive function of a normal healthy person.

MOUTH

• Food is chewed in the mouth and mixed with,

• Water

• Mucus

• Mineral salts

• Blood clotting factors

• Immunoglobulins,

• Lysozyme

• Enzyme: salivary amylase

This is an important first step in breaking down food.

PH levels in the mouth, are normally between, 5.4 to 7.5

CEPHALIC PHASE OF DIGESTION

Digestion is initiated by, the taste, sight, smell, and past experience of food, this stimulates the vagus nerves, to signal the stomach to begin releasing gastric juices.

The release of gastric juice begins before the food is even swallowed.

STOMACH

• This chime (food) then moves into the stomach, where it mixes with more of the following.

• Water

• Mucus, for lubrication, and protection of stomach lining.

• Mineral salts

• Hydrochloric acid from the Parietal cells, stops the action of salivary amylase, and acidifies the food, preventing microbes from multiplying, and provides an acid environment suitable for the pepsins to work.

• Pepsinogens from the chief cells, are activated by hydrochloric acid into pepsins and aided by pepsins already in the stomach.

• Intrinsic factor is also produced from the parietal cells, and helps carry B12 to the terminal ileum for absorption.

• The three muscle forms, (oblique, circular and longtitudonal smooth muscle) around the stomach churn the food to break it down.

• When no food has been eaten the resting PH in the pyloric antrum is around 3.5 to maintain an acidic environment in readiness for the arrival of food in the stomach.

• PH levels in the pyloric antrum should be within the parameters of 1.5 and 2, after food has been eaten and broken down in the stomach, and at this PH food is then passed to the digestive tract, and firstly the duodenum for further breakdown and absorption.

GASTRIC PHASE OF DIGESTION

So food has been ingested and is in the stomach.

When the acid levels in the pyloric antrum of the stomach rise above a PH of 3.5, the enteroendocrine cells in the pyloric antrum are triggered and release the hormone gastrin, into the blood, this initiates the release of breakdown of food in the stomach, and a continual cycle of breakdown of food in the stomach.

At a PH of 1.5 to 2 this acidic chime is squirted from the pyloric antrum through the pyloric sphincter, in small amounts at a time, into the Duodenum, where more enteroendocrine cells, in the duodenum, also release gastrin into the blood.

Gastrin in the blood, stimulates the stomach to release more gastric juices into the stomach. This phase ensures, that a continual cycle of breakdown of food in the stomach is continued, even after you have finished eating.

As food moves to the bottom of the stomach, it becomes more acidic until it reaches the pyloric antrum at a minimum PH of about 1.5 to 2, food at the top of the stomach is usually around a PH of 4 to 5.

If the food sensed by the enteroendocrine cells in the pyloric antrum and duodenum falls to a PH of around 1.5, then gastrin production is stopped, to prevent the environment in the stomach, pyloric antrum and duodenum, becoming too acidic.

INTESTINAL PHASE OF DIGESTION

When the food has passed into the duodenum and jejunum, more hormones are released by endocrine cells, these are in the form of the hormone complex, enterogastrone, this is made up of two hormones, secretin and cholecystokinin (CCK).

These hormones regulate gastric motility, to control the rate at which food enters the small intestine, this allows for more efficient digestion, and allows more time for bile from the liver, and juices from the pancreas, to mix with the food at the point of entry to the digestive tract, the sphincter of oddy, at the hepatopancreatic ampulla.

Cholecystokinin also stimulates the gallbladder to contract and release bile into the duodenum, the sphincter of oddi relaxes, due to a reflex action from the gallbladder contractions, it also stimulates the pancreas to release digestive enzymes precursors, and bicarbonates.

Secretin stimulates the secretion of bicarbonate, and enzyme precursors by the pancreas, but also inhibits the production of gastrin and acid in the stomach.

BREAKDOWN AND ABSORPTION

LIVER:

In the healthy intestine, between 500ml and 1000ml of bile should be produced every day.

Bile from the liver at a PH of 8, (vital for activation of pancreatic ases and gens) assists in raising intestinal food PH in the duodenum to 6.5 to 7.5 and consists of the following.

● Water

● Mineral salts

● Mucus

● Bile salts, SodiumTaurocholate and Sodium Glycocholate

● Bile pigments, mainly Bilirubin

● Cholesterol

PANCREAS

The pancreas secretes the following juices at a PH of around or just under 8.
This juice also assists in raising duodenal intestinal food PH TO 6.5 TO 7.5

● Water.

● Mineral salts.

● Lipase.

● Amylase

● Chymotrypsinogen

● Procarboxypeptidase.

● Trypsinogen

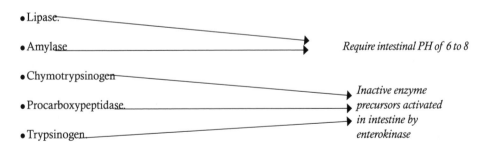

Require intestinal PH of 6 to 8

Inactive enzyme precursors activated in intestine by enterokinase

INTESTINE

Secretes juice with a PH of 7.8 to 8, also assists in raising intestinal food PH to 6.5 to 7.5

Intestinal juice contains the following

- Water.

- Mucus.

- Mineral salts.

- Enterokinase.

- Peptidase

- Lipase

- Sucrase

- Maltase

- Lactase

- Amylase

- Trypsin

Lipase and amylase from the pancreas, requiring an intestinal PH of 6 to 8, and aid in breaking down fats, and is aided by the bile salts sodium taurocholate, and sodium glycocholate from the liver, this makes fatty acids soluble, and able to be absorbed into the enterocytes and then into the lacteals of the villi.

Amylase from the pancreas requires an intestinal PH of 6 to 8, this aids in breaking down starches (polysaccharides) to disaccharides, and in turn, Sucrase, Maltase and Lactase aid in completing the breakdown of starches to monosaccarhides, before absorption into the enterocytes,

Trypsin and chymotrypsin are the activated form of the pancreatic secretions Trypsinogen and chymotrypsinogen, it is activated in the duodenum by enterokinase, trypsin breaks down polypeptides to tripeptides then dipeptides and in turn amino acids, it is aided in this process by Peptidase, this requires an optimum duodenal PH of 8, and a temperature of 37 °C to be activated, this will prove to be critical in the following explanation of digestive dysfunction.

Peptidases, in the enterocytes of the small intestine, from the pancreatic secretion procarboxypeptidase, requires an intestinal PH of at least 6 to be activated efficiently, mainly active in the enterocytes, and aids in breaking down peptides to amino acids, ready for absorption into the enterocytes.

BOWEL PH, ABSOLUTELY VITAL

BOWEL PH

This is absolutely vital for the correct functioning of the digestive tract, if the food in the Duodenum, and in particular at the point where food enters the duodenum, drops below a PH of 6, this can have serious consequences for the breakdown and absorption of food.

Bowel PH is directly influenced by four things, stomach PH, the production of pancreatic bicarbonates, the production of bile from the liver and digestive juices produced in the bowel.

Any coagulation within the liver, or any gallstones present in the gallbladder, leads to a lack of bile production and a reduction in the free flow of bile down the common bile duct, and a consequential drop in duodenal PH.

The Pancreas may be impinged upon, due to liver coagulation, or gallstones, this leads to a reduction in pancreatic bicarbonate and can further, and dramatically compound the problem, leading to a further reduction in PH in the duodenum.

Stomach PH plays a roll in duodenal PH, but this is only due to the compensation of the bowel, which will be discussed in the next section, Digestive Compensation.

Food from the stomach via the pyloric antrum and pyloric sphincter enters the duodenum at a PH of 1.5 to 3.5, if the liver and gallbladder are clogged this will impinge on the pancreas, and therefore not enough alkalising pancreatic bicarbonates will enter the food to raise the PH in the duodenum to the critical minimal PH of 6, to efficiently activate the pancreatic precursors, Trypsinogen, chymotrypsinogen and Procarboxypeptidase, this dramatically reduces the efficiency of the digestive tract to break down proteins to amino acids.

Lipases and Amylases, from the pancreas also require a minimal PH of 6, to work efficiently.

The more coagulation within the liver, or any gallstones present in the gallbladder or liver, can reduce the duodenal PH to as little as 5, this in turn can lead to serious consequences for the breakdown and absorption of proteins and fats, there will not be efficient activation of Pancreatic enzyme precursors, especially the ones involved in the breakdown of proteins.

Nutrients returning via the portal vein to the liver, are then dramatically reduced, especially amino acids, the liver will be short of amino acids, and therefore will have problems synthesising, and consequently the liver will become more and more dysfunctional, many enzymes, proteins, blood albumins, and building blocks of cells will be in short supply, other elements produced by the liver such as angiotensinogen may not be produced in sufficient quantities to fully regulate kidney functions, and peripheral functions related to homeostasis.

DIGESTIVE COMPENSATION

DIGESTIVE COMPENSATION STAGE 1, SWITCHING BETWEEN NORMAL BOWEL AND CONSTIPATION.

This is the first stage of digestive dysfunction, and often the first sign that a person is beginning to develop digestive problems.

These people are beginning to produce slightly less bile and pancreatic enzymes.

And bowel PH is beginning to fall.

These people can break down most foods, but if food containing high levels of protein and fat are consumed they begin to have a problems breaking them down, and compensation begins to occur. If they eat a light meal, such as a salad, fruit or vegetables they can break these foods down, and no observed digestive problems occur.

So what is happening in their digestive tract when they eat difficult to break down foods, such as steak pie, chips peas and gravy?

The food is taken down into their stomach and the gastric stage of digestion is initiated, it is triggered initially by chewing the food which signals the stomach that food is on its way, once the food is in the stomach hydrochloric acid and pepsins begin to break down the food.

As the PH begins to fall to around 1 to 1.5 the pyloric valve opens and begins to squirt food into the Duodenum, the gastrin released into the blood from the enteroendocrine cells in the duodenum ensures a continuous cycle of breakdown in the stomach, but this is where we encounter our first problem, because the liver is slightly clogged and there is some impingement of the pancreas, reduced levels of bicarbonates bile and enzymes are passed into the duodenum and therefore the PH in the duodenum is unable to rise to the optimum 6.5 to 7.5, and can be as low as 5.5 to 6, this is too acidic and consequently poor activation of pancreatic enzyme precursors ensues, and the ability to break down proteins into amino acids is reduced.

The enteroendocrine cells in the duodenum then sense the lower than optimum PH and gastrin secretion by the duodenum is then reduced, therefore the gastric cycle is interrupted and food is kept in the stomach for a longer period of time, and gastrin released by the stomach continues the processes in the stomach.

But the gastrin in the stomach only continues being produced at a reduced level, in a healthy person the food in the stomach is normally more acidic in the pyloric antrum, and less acidic at the fundus, but in this scenario food is churned for much longer and the entire contents of the stomach become more acidic, and the acid is dissipated throughout the stomach, the PH in the pyloric antrum will now be slightly higher than normal, where it would usually be, 1 to 1.5 it will be around 2, to 2.5 but higher up in the stomach at the fundus, the PH will be lower than normal, (too acidic), 2 to 2.5 due to the lack of continual transgression of food passing from the stomach, and dissipation of acid within the stomach.

Now when the food is squirted into the duodenum it is at a slightly higher PH than the norm, 2 to 2.5, and although the liver is slightly clogged and impinges on the pancreas, the amount of bicarbonates, bile and enzymes passed by the liver and pancreas can raise duodenal PH to 6 to 7 ensuring more effective breakdown of proteins and fats, even though the PH in the duodenum is slightly reduced.

The inactive enzyme precursors chymotripsinogen, procarboxypeptidase, and tripsinogen can now be activated effectivelyin the duodenum by enterokinase, and lipase and amylase are still able to work effectively.

Note that the lower PH in the duodenum is detected on the initial squirt of food into duodenum from the pyloric antrum, if the PH in the duodenum is unable to be lifted to 6.5 to 7.5 then compensation is initiated, this usually only takes about twenty minutes after eating food, only a very slight shift in duodenal PH, from the normally attainable 6.5 to 7.5 down to a duodenal PH of around 6 to 7 is enough to trigger compensation.

The next compensatory process then takes place in the digestive tract, and involves peristalsis, secretin and cholecystokinin when combined form the hormone complex enterogastrone.

Normally when food passes into the duodenum the intestinal phase is triggered, and enterogastrone is produced to regulate motility and the transgression of food from the stomach, when compensation begins to occur slightly more enterogastrone is produced slowing down the compensatory process slightly more then would be the norm.

Cholecystokinin triggers the gallbladder to contract and secretin triggeres the pancreas to release enzyme precursors, and this action in turn trigger's a reflex action which signals the hepatopancreatic sphincter to relax, allowing flow of liver and pancreatic elements to enter the food in the duodenum.

There is an extremely fine balance in the relationship between gastrin and enterogastrone, if the food in the duodenum cannot be raised to the correct PH, then enterogastrone will try to regulate the motility of food from the stomach, even if this means leaving food in the stomach for many hours before it is in a position to break it down in the duodenum.

One of the most noticeable changes in the intestine is in relation to peristalsis, when compensation stage one begins to occur, the PH in the bowel is very slightly lower than would be considered the norm, therefore to allow more time to extract nutrients from the steak pie chips peas and gravy the person has just eaten, peristalsis will slow down slightly, this will allow more time for the intestinal juices, enterokinase (enteropeptidase), peptidases, mineral salts, mucus, water, lipase, sucrase, maltase and lactase to effectively break down the foods in the intestine.

In stage one compensation the absorptive pattern of the villi and enterocytes does not appear to be affected, and absorption is maintained very close to what would be considered normal, with no adverse effects occurring in transfer of nutrients to the portal vein, blood and lymph.

Digestive compensation stage one has just begun to take place.

SYMPTOMS OF DIGESTIVE COMPENSATION STAGE 1

If a meal which is difficult to break down has been eaten, this patient will now feel slightly bloated in their stomach, with indigestion and constipation.

Energy levels are usually still maintained in stage one, and often the patient does not present with obvious symptoms.

People often self prescribe at this stage and may take OTC antacids and laxatives, to try and alleviate their symptoms, and do not feel the need to visit their doctor.

These symptoms do need attention, but if antacids are taken it will interfere with compensation stage 1, they will feel better for taking antacids, with less reflux, but they will impede their ability to extract many vitamins and minerals, and after a few months or even years they will begin to feel weak and tired, it is often at this stage that they visit their doctor, and are given even stronger antacids or acid blockers, this further interrupts their absorbtive pattern, and actually compounds the problem.
Prescribing laxatives for constipation totally unhinges compensation and leaves the patient even less able to extract nutrients.

This is the beginning of a slippery slope for the patient, digestive compensation was trying to extract nutrients in a failing digestive environment, and these drugs completely interfere with these compensatory processes.

These patients don't require drugs, in the first instance they require a dietary change, and once their digestive function has stabilised, their liver and pancreatic function can be recovered with liver flushes, if this course of action is undertaken at this relatively early stage in digestive dysfunction, the prognosis is excellent and the patient will make a full recovery.

DIGESTIVE COMPENSATION STAGE 2, SWITCHING BETWEEN CONSTIPATION AND LOOSE BOWELS.

We have already established why constipation takes place, as discussed in the previous explanation "digestive compensation stage 1".

The following will explain my understanding of what is happening when you begin to switch between constipation and loose bowels.

In stage 2, if easy to break down foods are eaten, such as salad, then the patient will have constipation, whereas in stage 1 they had normal bowel movement, in stage 2 digestive compensation takes place even if easy to break down foods are eaten, this is due to an inability to pass enough bile and enzymes to raise intestinal PH.

If very difficult to break down food such as, steak pie, chips peas and gravy are eaten in stage 2 then the patient will have loose bowels, whereas in stage one compensation they would have constipation.

In this scenario food has been retained in the stomach for much longer, as described in digestive compensation stage 1, but because the liver has become more clogged with the possible presence of gallstones, this will have impinged on the pancreas to a greater degree, there are even less bicarbonates available to aid in raising duodenal PH to the optimum 6.5 to 7.5.

If duodenal PH is unable to be raised above 5.5 to 6, then further compensatory processes are initiated, enterogastrone continues to regulate gastric motility, as in stage 1, when food is passed from the stomach to the duodenum, the PH is at 2 to 2.5, as in stage 1, but due to a lack of ability to raise duodenal PH above 5.5 to 6 changes in intestinal motility are initiated, peristaltic sequencing begins to speed up, or slow down, depending on whether easy or hard to break down food has been eaten.

Peristalsis cannot slow down to a speed below stage 1, where constipation is triggered, otherwise intestinal motility would stop, this would inevitably end in death, so nature has evolved a trick to alleviate this problem if difficult to break down foods are eaten, compensation stage 2 then initiates the speeding up of intestinal peristalsis to a rate faster than would be conventionally considered the norm, this speeded up peristalsis has profound consequences for extraction and absorption of nutrients in the intestine, but at least the patient will still be alive.

By far the greatest problem is the low PH in the bowel, the intestine has to try and regulate to some degree this acidic environment, and at the same time extract some nutrients. Enterogastrone (cholecystokinin and secretin) are produced in larger amounts to try and pass as much bile and enzymes into the food as possible.

Therefore more compensatory processes are initiated within the bowel, much more water, mucus and mineral salts are released into the bowel, this is to try and raise intestinal PH to at least 6 to 6.5 as food passes through the intestine, the problem is that in stage 2 compensation the PH in the duodenum is especially effected, and if the patients symptoms are carefully observed, it becomes clear that poor breakdown and absorption of B Vitamins is taking place.

If gallstones are present then the continual contractions of the gallbladder, which are triggered by cholecystokinin can cause pain, or at least discomfort after a difficult meal has been eaten, and consequently the reflex action controlling hepatopancreatic sphincter function is constantly activated, this is also a compensatory process to ensure as much bile and enzymes can enter the duodenum as possible.

Enterokinase (enteropeptidase) is produced in copious amounts by microvilli in the intestine, this is to try and activate as many of the enzyme precursors chymotrypsinogen, procarboxypeptidase, tripsinogen as possible, but due to the continual low PH, there is inefficient activation and therefore proteins are not broken down to polypeptides, peptides efficiently, and due to the upset PH the enterocytes of the villi are affected and poor conversion to amino acids ensues.

Because there is impairment of liver function, less sodium taurocholate and sodium glycholate are passed into the duodenum, therefore emulsification of fats is impaired and in turn lipase in the bowel and enterocytes does not complete the breakdown of fats to fatty acids and glycerol efficiently, and consequentially poor uptake of fatty acids is able to take place in the lacteals, and taken up in lymph.

Sucrase, maltase and lactase are the least effected elements in the intestine, and consequently uptake of sugars is the least affected part of absorption.

This pauses a problem in itself, people who have clogging of the liver are almost invariably addicted to sugar, usually chocolate, this is because the patient is obtaining most of their energy from carbohydrate, and are unable to efficiently break down oils and fat.

Their overconsumption of carbohydrates can further affect pancreatic function, compounding their digestive issues further.

Bilirubin the by product of breakdown of erythrocytes is converted to stercobilin in the large intestine, this is responsible for colouring the stool and also deodorises faeces, therefore if the patient has light coloured foul smelling stools, it indicates poor liver function and also poor microbal activity in the intestine.

The intestinal mucosa begins to degrade further over time, this will be discussed in stage three compensation.

SYMPTOMS OF DIGESTIVE COMPENSATION STAGE 2

Stage 2 compensation presents with many more symptoms, than stage 1.

The patient will present with most or all of the following symptom, and has usually been diagnosed as having IBS.

- Switching between loose bowels and constipation

- Often addicted to sugary products, usually chocolate

- Hungry most of the time.

- Bloating of the stomach.

- Acid reflux, (severe in some cases).

- A lack of energy.

- Sensitivity to bright lights.

- General tiredness (bordering on ME).

- Disrupted sleep patterns.

- General aching of joints, especially knees and shoulders.

- Lower back ache.

- Lethargy

- Tinea pedis (athletes foot)

- Fungal toenails

- Anxiety

- Sleep not beneficial

- Haemorrhoids (piles)

- Dead limbs when sleeping

- Tingling in fingers and toes.

CONDITIONS RELATING TO DIGESTIVE COMPENSATION STAGE 2.

- IBS.

- Celiac disease (possibly, more likely in stage 3 compensation, the emergency state)

- Diverticulitis.

- Crohns disease, possibly at terminal ileum, with B12 pernicious Anaemia.

- Helicobacter pylori.

- Intussusception

- Ulcerative colitis.

- Gastric or duodenal ulcers.

- Myalgic encephalitis.

- Colonitis.

- Iron deficient anaemia.

- Aesophogitis.

This stage of digestive dysfunction can be much more challenging to recover, long term use of antacids and acid blockers will have severely interfered with absorptive pathways for many years, this will have caused degradation of the digestive tract and many organs of the body, and more clogging of the liver, in turn impinging on the pancreas, and also affecting kidney function.

The practitioner will have to work closely with the patient to encourage them to change their diet and flush the liver, some dedication is required on the part of the patient, they must adhere to quite a strict dietary regime, and maybe two or three years of liver flushes to fully recover their digestive function.

DIGESTIVE COMPENSATION STAGE 3, (THE EMERGENCY STATE), PERMANENT LOOSE BOWELS.

Compensation stage 3 can be quite serious, very poor breakdown and absorption of food takes place in the digestive tract, many foods such as nuts, carrots, corn, seeds, pass through the digestive tract with little or no attempt to break them down in the digestive tract.

In advanced stage three compensation, (the emergency state) it does not matter what the patient eats, even simple foods cannot be broken down without triggering full compensation, These patients never revert to constipation, as in stage 2 compensation, but have permanent loose bowels all the time.

In this scenario all the previously described compensatory factors of stage 2 are present, triggering permanent loose bowels, but in stage 3 compensation there are also additional factors relating to the mucosa of the bowel and the villi, lacteals, enterocytes, plus the added complication of poor recycling of fluids from both the small and large intestine.

After a few months or even years of permanent loose bowels the digestive mucosa is usually affected, epithelial goblet cells begin to be affected and secrete less protective mucus around the lumen of the intestine, villi become less permeable and can become flattened (celiac disease), initially much more fluids, water, mucus, mineral salts are released into the bowel to try and raise the PH to protective levels, villi become affected and even if they are not flattened, as in celiac disease, the ability of the enterocytes to extract nutrients through the villi and microvilli is very much impeded, and therefore very few vitamins and minerals enter the capillaries, patients fulfilling this criteria are just as intolerant to wheat as a celiac, have difficulty breaking down proteins, and are also far less able to break down and absorb oils and fats.

The aforementioned dictates that no one person can be soley intolerant to one food, if you are wheat intolerant then you also have to be intolerant to other foods, the ensuing change in gut flora, and the balance of good and bad bacteria in the gut causes other reactions to take place, when food intolerants are in stage 3 their gut flora becomes so imbalanced that if sugars are eaten in too large a quantity, as in milk lactose, oranges, processed sugar, or many gluten free products available in supermarkets, the bad bacteria multiplies very rapidly causing extreme wind, bloating and intestinal discomfort, intestinal pains are often experienced, due to peristaltic waves desperately trying to evacuate the bowel, whilst regaining some degree of ability to extract some nutrients.

Uptake of nutrients from the entire intestine is poor, and therefore returning nutrients vitamins and minerals via the portal vein to the liver are in short supply, and therefore due to impaired villi and enterocyte activity and permeability the taking of replacement supplements is virtually a waste of time and money, this leaves the liver very little to work with, this compounds the problem impinging further on the pancreas, a vicious circle can then ensue, and in the case of the celiac condition, (flattened villi), if diagnosis is not ascertained, death can even occur.

Uptake of lipids into the lymphatic system are impeded further reducing nutrient supply, Peyers patches and general lymphatic activity may then be affected.

The entire bowel will now be too acidic, if this scenario persists for a long period of time the lining of the bowel can become degraded, columnar epithelial tissue can become degraded, muscle layers throughout the digestive tract can become weakened, this breakdown of tissues can lead to, diverticulitis, crohns disease, ulcerative colitis, gastric and duodenal ulcers, and other digestive issues.

As gut permeability continues to progressively become more chronic, many nutrients are malabsorbed, toxins are produced and can now build up in the intestine, some of them can pass into the lymph and capillaries, this in turn can enter the blood, as this circulates around the body it can make the patient feel quite ill, fluey, extremely tired, headaches, feeling spaced out, memory function can often be affected, stiff joints, stiff muscles, spasmodic skin palpitations, involuntary muscle spasms.
This scenario in alternative medicine circles is commonly referred to as leaky gut syndrome.

In stage 3, digestive function is virtually out of control, but usually the patient has learnt consciously or subconsciously that certain foods affect them, they know that if they eat things like bread they are worse, often they change their diet slightly, and their digestive tract can just cope, and although they still have some discomfort they are able to function on a daily basis.

Others completely collapse and find that working is impossible, they have a chronic condition and find little relief from their symptoms, and if conventional drug protocols are undertaken the prognosis is very poor, often after a number of years bowel resections are undertaken, or other surgery on their digestive tract is required to stabilise their condition.

SYMPTOMS OF DIGESTIVE COMPENSATION STAGE 3

- People in the advanced stages of stage 3 are very weak, and often take to their beds for most of the day.

- Bloating of stomach.

- Permanent loose bowels.

- Extreme exhaustion, (possible myalgic encephalitis, not immune related)

- Foul smelling faeces.

- Light coloured stools.

- Eyes affected by bright lights.

- Aching shoulders.

- Aching muscles.

- Aching knees.

- Headaches.

- Extreme flatulence.

- Poor name memory.

- Poor attention span.

- Tired but cannot sleep.

- Disturbed sleep patterns.

- Acid reflux.

CONDITIONS RELATING TO DIGESTIVE COMPENSATION STAGE 3

- IBS.

- Celiac disease.

- Crohns disease.

- Diverticulitis.

- Helicobacter pylori

- Intussusception

- Myalgic encephalitis.(not immune related)

- B12 pernicious anaemia.

- Iron deficient anaemia

- Tinea pedis.

- Candida albicans.

- Ulcerative colitis.

- Haemorrhoids.

- Colonitis

- Aesophogitis (caused by reflux)

TREATMENTS

CONVENTIONAL TREATMENT PROTOCOLS

It is important to understand that people with even minor digestive problems, such as bloating and indigestion are beginning to loose their ability to break down food, and their digestive system is beginning to compensate.

With conventional treatment these people may initially be given antacids, this in the short term gives them some relief from their indigestion and bloating, but this course of action further interferes with digestive processes, and because compensation has been imbalanced some nutrients which were being broken down and absorbed before taking antacids are now far less able to be broken down and absorbed.

It may take a few months or even a year or so, but these people usually very slowly get returning symptoms, the underlying cause of their problem is that their liver and pancreas are not working efficiently, therefore taking antacids is only treating symptoms and not addressing the cause of their problems.

It is vital that a patient with prolonged acid reflux and bloating initially changes their diet, they need to eat foods, which they can still break down, without tripping their digestive tract into compensation.

If this protocol is undertaken recourse to using antacids or acid blockers is not necessary, and the patient will observe a dramatic change in their symptoms within two weeks.

In virtually all cases of a patient passing through a doctors surgery presenting with acid reflux, the first course of action is to prescribe antacids, tagamet, losec, etc, the ball is now rolling and the clock is ticking on the countdown to further problems developing in the future, as less and less nutrients are broken down and absorbed the liver and pancreas, and indeed all the organs related to digestion are very slowly further degraded.

From the moment you first begin to take antacids your bowel PH will never be correct, an acidic bowel will be the end result as compensation within the digestive tract is unable to take place as nature intended.

The consequential incorrect PH within the bowel will over time begin to cause other problems to develop, the walls of the bowel begin to break down due to incorrect PH, this I have seen in virtually every case I have dealt with, I have taken a life history of hundreds of patients and in almost every case they follow the same pattern of bowel degredation, patients may go on to develop any of the following conditions, diverticulitis, ulcerative colitis, crohns disease, duodenal or gastric ulcers, pernicious anaemia, iron deficiency, and even bowel cancer.

Conventional treatment protocol then moves on to more drugs, anti-inflammatories, protein pump inhibitors, etc. this again is treating symptoms, these conditions would not have developed if in the first instance a dietary change and liver flushes were initially undertaken.

If dietary changes are not undertaken and liver flushes not completed these patients progress further into more serious scenarios, where invasive procedures may be required, such as a bowel resection.

Parasitic, bacterial or fungal infections may have taken hold if the patient is in stage three compensation, (the emergency state), and in severe cases may need to be treated with antibiotics, or other drugs, to kill off the infection, but I have to say that the use of antibiotics should only be used as the very last resort, and if used should be targeted and not broadband antibiotics, they will disrupt the gut flora even further, and leave the patient even less able to break down the foods they eat.

Other complications may include vitamin B12 deficiency, often this is due to Crohns disease, and damage to the small intestine around the terminal ileum, where B12 is absorbed, often people with serious digestive issues who are in the digestive compensation stage 3 (the emergency state) scenario, don't produce enough intrinsic factor and therefore are unable to carry B12 to the terminal ileum for absorption.

This leaves them with pernicious anaemia, and B12 injections are required to stabilise RBC maturation issues.

This situation does not usually occur with people in stage one or two of compensation, they are usually in stage three before developing B12 deficiencies.

Iron deficient anaemia is often an issue even in stage one of compensation, people often report taking iron supplements for years and eventually are diagnosed with IBS or Celiac disease, the lack of iron leaves them weak and tired, and due to the fact that these people have a very poor absorption pattern, their iron levels only rise slightly when iron supplements are prescribed.

They begin to absorb iron again if a dietary change is undertaken, and as long as they are eating foods which they can still break down, which will not trip them into digestive compensation.

Many nutrients, vitamins and minerals are also very poorly absorbed once digestive compensation takes place, patently if you do not have sufficient iron or VitaminB12 then you are not going to extract and absorb many other elements in sufficient quantities to maintain homeostasis within the entire body.

This point is so often overlooked by the medical faternity, but even if supplement vitamins and minerals are prescribed there will be very little uptake of these due to poor digestive function, if supplements are taken you must regain significant digestive function before obvious signs and changes may be observed in the individual.

Often people are wasting their money taking supplements, they may as well throw their money down the toilet, because that is where most of the supplements end up.

After digestive function has been recovered the individual does not require supplements, because they will be extracting and absorbing more efficiently anyway, there are only a couple of exemptions to this rule. Due to intensive agriculture elements such as selenium and especially zinc are so depleted in our soils that very little is found in food, zinc especially is vital for correct digestive function, so often I will prescribe zinc throughout recovery, and even small amounts after recovery.

IMPORTANT NOTE

It has to be understood, that the first, and vital initial approach to digestive dysfunction, is to change the fuel that the patient is putting in their mouth, and not to reach straight into the drugs cabinet.

If a dietary change does not alleviate symptoms, then further investigation may be undertaken, endoscopy, colonoscopy, blood tests, faecal tests etc.

OBSERVED COMPLICATIONS

DIABETES

Storage capacity for glycogen can be impeded due to the LIVER being clogged, and inefficiencies can occur in the regulation of blood sugars, due to inefficiencies in the production of glucagon, and insulin by the pancreas, when the liver is coagulated, there is impingement on the Alpha, and Beta cells in the pancreas, because the supply of nutrients required to keep these cells functioning effectively can be in short supply.

If people are in the emergency state within the bowel, (permanent loose bowels) then their digestive tract will be more porous, and inefficiencies in the absorption of glucose will overload the pancreas further, glucose will drop into the blood very quickly, causing potential hyper and hypo blood sugar levels, the pancreas has to work very hard to regulate blood sugar levels once the liver has become clogged.

Many people with the inability to breakdown food are virtually addicted to sugary products, this is because their body in the main is having to supply energy from carbohydrate alone, because they are having problems breaking down proteins, and oils and fats. This puts stress on the pancreas every day, and can eventually lead to failure of the islets of langerhans.

Storage capacity within the liver is very much impeded if the liver is clogged, therefore there is less capacity for glycogen storage, this creates a problem when large amounts of carbohydrate are consumed, the pancrease has to continually produce insulin to try and store blood glucose.

This over production of insulin can eventually cause over compensation, and too much insulin production on a daily basis, so that when carbohydrate has not been eaten for a few hours, a hypoglycaemic condition can ensue, and blood glucose levels may fall to as little as 2 to 4 mmol/litre, leaving the person feeling weak and shaky, I myself had this scenario, and observed it in other people, after testing their blood glucose levels, throughout their recovery.

This is often referred to as a pre diabetic state, eventually the pancreas can become degraded if this level of insulin production has to be maintained, and eventually it will reach a point of degradation and exhaustion where insufficient quantities of insulin are produced, and the person then begins to develop type two diabetes, (hyperglycaemia)

Other problems may occur, often there is restriction at the hepatopancreatic sphincter, this restriction is often caused because the gallbladder is degraded, has stones in it, or may even be calcified to some degree. If these scenarios are present the gall bladder tries to contracts, but inefficiencies occur, this interferes with the reflex response to the hepatopancreatic sphincter, and thus very poor control of dilation of the hepatopancreatic sphincter can ensue, this can inhibit the free flow of pancreatic juices, and of course bile, if this situation ensues for a long period of time then it can damage the pancreas.

More importantly if any of the Gens, such as chymotripsinogen, trypsinogen or Procarboxypeptidase are activated within the pancreas, damage to the alpha and beta cells will occur, consequently insulin and glucagon production will be impeded, and a diabetic state will ensue.

As I progressed through recovery I was completing liver and gallbladder flushes at regular intervals, I was constantly recording my blood glucose levels, and was surprised to find that after every flush my blood glucose levels began to rise slightly.

When I was at my worst, as I began this recovery programme, my blood glucose levels were consistently around 2, but after each liver and gallbladder flush my blood glucose levels began to rise, after full recovery I now maintain blood glucose levels of 4.5 to 6, this is considered normal, I am quite convinced that if I had not recovered my digestive tract, I would now be a diabetic.

Others I have followed through recovery have also followed exactly the same patterns of blood glucose stabilisation, this confirms to me that liver coagulation has a dramatic affect on the stability of the whole digestive tract, and many other organs of the body, these includes the endocrine system of which the pancreas is a part, poor breakdown and absorption of food requires compensation to take place, to maintain stability within the body, in this case the pancreas has to try and work harder with less available nutrients, therefore, eventually, cell degradation can occurs within the pancreas, but if the liver and gallbladder flushes are undertaken, the pancreas can regain its efficiency, and fully recover its normal function.

RENIN, ANGIOTENSINOGEN, A.C.E, AND FEELING COLD

I could not regulate my body temperature when in the depths of my food intolerance, and after devising an experiment to monitor my body temperature, and studying rennin, angiotensinogen, aldosterone, may have found the reason why I could not regulate body temperature efficiently.

To try and work out why I was cold when sedentary, and sweat when doing very little exercise, I devised an experiment to measure my core temperature, compared or relative to my peripheral temperature, this revealed some interesting results.

In the depths of food intolerance I measured my core temperature with a thermometer in my mouth and anus, and my peripheral temperature with thermometers in the closed inner elbow of my right arm and a thermometer in my hand.

I repeatedly over five years throughout my recovery sat outside in an ambient temperature of 2 to 7 deg C, with the same amount of clothing on, for 30 minutes. I repeated this many times over the five years of recovery to see if there were any measurable changes in the results.

When I was at my worst, my peripheral temperature dropped rapidly from 37°C to as low as 33°C. I found my core temperature dropped from 37°C to 35.5°C at which point I was shivering violently and ended the experiment.

But interestingly for the first twenty minutes my core temperature was following my peripheral temperature down in parallel, therefore I could only ascertain that peripheral vasoconstriction was not taking place efficiently.

As I progressed through my recovery I repeated the same experiments, and found that my peripheral temperature dropped off more rapidly, but my core temperature only dropped off very slowly, there was a definite differential between the rate of peripheral temperature drop and core temperature drop, there was a marked difference between the results of the experiments, before and after recovery.

Patently peripheral vasoconstriction was taking place much more markedly after recovery, so I began to try and find any possible reasons why.

After studying homeostasis I began to realise that there was a link between the liver and vasoconstriction, the LIVER produces Angiotensinogen, if the liver is coagulated there is a distinct possibility that there may be inefficient production of Angiotensinogen, if this is the case then rennin released by the kidneys could have less angiotensinogen to interact with, therefore there could be less angiotensin 1 produced.

Even if you produce the correct amount of angiotensinogen, there could still be a problem converting it.

because angiotensin converting enzyme, from the lungs and proximal convoluted tubules in the kidneys, would produce very little angiotensin 2, why? Because ACE is an enzyme, and if the LIVER is clogged, you cannot break down proteins to amino acids efficiently, therefore the amino acids would be in short supply, consequently enzyme production would be low, so less angiotensin converting enzyme may be available, compounding the problem.

So due to the fact that there may be less angiotensinogen, and angiotensing converting enzyme available, there could be very little angiotensin 2, and therefore poor vaso constriction.

This would explain why I found a differential in my falling peripheral / core body temperature results after recovery, but very little differential in my falling peripheral / core body temperature before recovery.

After recovery I could be producing more angiotensinogen from the LIVER, and more enzymes would be available to make angiotensin converting enzyme, therefore vasoconstriction would take place more efficiently.

In the depths of intolerance there may be a very slightly reduced production of angiotensinogen, or ACE and therefore very little vasoconstriction, and little differential between peripheral and core temperature as the body cooled.

These scenarios are only subtle and not life threatening, but are chronic, long term problems, in a food intolerant person.

This may explain why food intolerants often feel cold, and quickly freeze, if sedentary.

This would explain why I now feel much warmer in general, I am often stood with people who say "its cold today isn't it", and I say to myself no not really, I feel quite warm, my core temperature is obviously being maintained very close to 37 degrees, but my periferal temperature drops quite markedly, if someone touches my skin they say I feel cold, but I don't feel cold myself.

I am obviously breaking down food more efficiently now, after full recovery, therefore I am burning more fuel, and can maintain core temperature stability far more effectively, and also run the systems relating to homeostasis at their optimum.

There may also be a link to the amount of Aldosterone available, and possibly the reasons why people feel weak and tired in the depths of Food intolerance, this will be explained in the next section.

RENAL HORMONAL FLOW

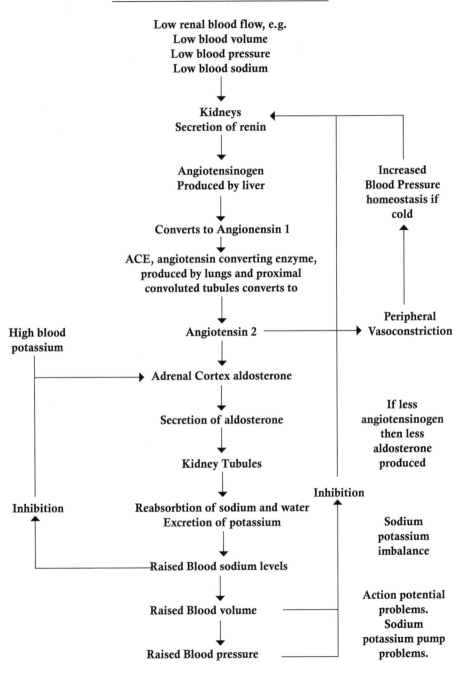

Low renal blood flow, e.g.
Low blood volume
Low blood pressure
Low blood sodium

↓

Kidneys
Secretion of renin

↓

Angiotensinogen
Produced by liver

Increased
Blood Pressure
homeostasis if
cold

↓

Converts to Angionensin 1

↓

ACE, angiotensin converting enzyme,
produced by lungs and proximal
convoluted tubules converts to

↓

Peripheral
Vasoconstriction

Angiotensin 2 ———→

High blood
potassium

↓

→ Adrenal Cortex aldosterone

↓

Secretion of aldosterone

If less
angiotensinogen
then less
aldosterone
produced

↓

Kidney Tubules

↓

Inhibition

Inhibition

Reabsorbtion of sodium and water
Excretion of potassium

Sodium
potassium
imbalance

↓

Raised Blood sodium levels

↓

Raised Blood volume ———

Action potential
problems.
Sodium
potassium pump
problems.

↓

Raised Blood pressure ———

ALDOSTERONE ANGIOTENSINOGEN AND FEELING WEAK, ME SYMPTOMS

The adrenals become degraded due to lack of nutrient availability, exhaustion of the adrenal glands is mainly due to the pressure they have been under, over the preceding years, whilst their digestive tract has been compensating, and overloading the adrenals, causing them to produce copious amounts of adrenalin and noradrenalin to try and maintain energy through over stimulation, relying on the person running in fright and flight mode instead of normal hormonal regulation.

Na +(sodium) and k+(potassium) and action potentials ?, below is a possible explanation of weakness due to insufficiencies in hormone production, by the adrenals and LIVER.

If less angiotensinogen is produced by the LIVER, due to coagulation, then as has been previously discussed, and highlighted in the flow chart, there may be less aldosterone produced.

This will lead to very poor reabsorption of sodium and water, and a build up in potassium, this is bourne out by observing the symptoms of patients who have food intolerance, and digestive compensation.

They usually pass a normal amount of water when in the depths of food intolerance, but they are often retentive, and look like Michelin man, this may be due to a lack of blood albumins, which is discussed in the next section, but when they are first put on the recovery diet, they pass very large amounts of water, for about a month, this is probably because their kidneys have less toxic load to deal with, and the liver begins to produce more blood albumins, altering osmotic pressure and releasing copious amounts of water, which is passed through the kidneys, this uncovers another problem which was being masked by digestive compensation, whilst in the depths of food intolerance.

When they are passing large amounts of water, Na+ is taken out along with the water due to a poor production of aldosterone, K+ levels will be high relative to Na+, the adrenal gland should sense this, and trigger aldosterone production, but the adrenals are usually exhausted after years of digestive compensation, and maybe cannot respond properly and produce enough Aldosterone to regulate Na+, water, and K+. This scenario compounds the problem when associated with a very slightly reduced production of angiotensinogen from the LIVER.

Therefore a fractional imbalance in K+ and Na+ ensues, this is not life threatening but is a subtle enough change to upset the action potential in neurons, and poor transmission of impulses down the neurons, the synapses could also be affected, due to a slightly reduced supply of neurotransmitters, these will also be in short supply, due to inefficient absorption of cations such as calcium, added to this acetylcholine production will also be affected, leaving the patient with weak muscles, due to poor neuron and synapse activation.

This often manifests itself as M.E, yuppie flu, (myalgic encephalitis), and often people are wrongly diagnosed with this condition. Their problem is a clogged liver and not an immune disorder or a dormant virus from years past, which the body has failed to eradicate properly.

Originally I thought that it was a lack of ADH causing problems with fluid balance, but the anterior pituitary gland does not appear to be implicated in other systemic hormonal related problems, so it is unlikely to be causing problems in relation to fluid balance, and the kidneys appear to respond to stimulus if an aldosterone stimulant is administered in the form of the herb, liquorice (glycyrrhiza glabra), this herb can also produce ACTH activity, and is vital in recovering the adrenal cortex, and adrenal function.

When Liquorice herb is administered a definite response occurs, and antidiuretic activity is observed in the individual, muscle strength usually begins to recover, and other symptoms such as muscle cramps, paresthesias (numbness of fingers, tingling), involuntary muscle twitching, skin palpitations, and in severe cases, nausea and even heart palpitations begin to disappear.

In effect these individuals have had hyperkalemia and hyponatremia, but not to life threatening degrees, subtle changes are involved, and maybe the parameters recognised as being the norm in intracellular and blood $Na+$ and $K+$ levels should be studied and re evaluated testing people with food intolerances, this may give us a better understanding of the subtle changes involved which cause problems to occur.

Using the herb liquorice indicates that ADH is not involved, but most of the problems are with angiotensinogen, adrenal insufficiency, and aldosterone production, because $Na+$ and $K+$ are patently involved and imbalanced, liquorice stimulates more production of these hormones, the reaction and changed state of the individual after the administration of Liquorice, is similar to that of treating a patient with liquorice when they have Addisons disease, where a marked improvement is also observed.

At the end of the day many of these problems can be traced back to insufficiencies within the LIVER.

SODIUM POTASSIUM PUMP

If there is only a fractional Na+ and K+ imbalance then every cell in the body is affected by it, intracellular and extracellular balance is upset in people with food intolerances, this is brought on by a clogged liver, low levels of extra cellular sodium, can lead to peripheral oedema in people before they adopt the recovery diet, after adopting the diet compensatory ADH levels drop off, and then we are left with a lack of aldosterone production.

At this stage peripheral oedema diminishes, but we are still left with a very slight shift in the ability to move Na+ and K+ across cell membranes, and therefore the environment within all cells is not conducive to healthy cell activity.

Other problems also occur, due to the lack of amino acid, enzyme and protein activity brought about by a clogged liver, protein receptor channels on all cells of the body may be slightly compromised, and therefore compounding problems with the balance of Na+ and K+, these protein channels on cells are required to pump Na+ and K+ against their concentration gradients, to allow correct balance at an intracellular and an extracellular level.

CONCLUSION

The previously described section on issues regarding angiotensinogen, aldosterone, Ma+ K+, sodium potassium pump etc, are very complex problems, and many other aspects can affect stability in these processes.

But the aspect covered here are possibly the main contributory factors, and failures associated with food intolerance and a clogged liver. To go into detail about all aspects regarding renal imbalances would fill a book in itself, so I have filtered it down, and concentrated on the more serious aspects which require treatment during recovery.

But if these problems are addressed a vast improvement is observed in the individual, although I have to say that fluid imbalances are notoriously bad to treat and recover.

It only takes a fractional shift in the balance of electrolytes to initiate slight changes in the appearance of the individual, often giving them a slightly retentive appearance in stage 2 compensation, and Michelin man appearance in stage 3 compensation, (the emergency state)

RHEUMATIC SYMPTOMS

Rheumatic symptoms usually occur in patients in stages 2 and 3 of compensation, this mainly affects synovial joints, this is possibly due initially to a poor ability to maintain cartilage, and synovial fluid being affected by lack of nutrients, brought on by poor intestinal absorption.

Virtually all patients in stages 2 and 3 of compensation will have joint ache, especially of the knees, lower back and shoulders. These scenarios begin to dissipate once their diet is changed and recovery is under way.

These are definite observations in all people with digestive problems, I cannot unravel the complex processes involved in these rheumatic problems, but I do know this, absolute changes are observed in the individual within five to eight weeks of starting the recovery diet and programme.

These individuals are not presenting with rheumatoid arthritis, with inflamed joints, or osteo arthritic signs, but do have definite rheumatic problems.

I myself had synovial joint ache, this began to improve once I adopted the diet. I was then left with the lower back pain until I finally cleaned my liver, at which point my back improved dramatically, I still get back ache but I am sure this is due to mechanical issues, and a probable prolapsed disc, I still have numbness in superficial peroneal (musculocutaneous) dermatome of my right lower leg, this would relate to where my lower back ache eminates from, at L4, 5, S1.

BLOOD ALBUMINS

When in the depths of food intolerance, and clogging of the liver, it may be causing malfunction of the cells involved in producing blood albumins, these are proteins synthesised from amino acids, but intolerants do not break down proteins to amino acids efficiently, therefore the amino acid pool may low, and the liver has less amino acids to work with resulting in very slight imbalances in blood albumin levels.

Until a food intolerants diet is changed, there is poor breakdown of proteins, but once their diet is changed, light easily digested proteins, such as fish and chicken are digested more efficiently, more proteins, and thus amino acids are then present via the portal vein for the liver to synthesise into blood albumins.

This increase in blood albumins, coupled with the previously discussed Na+ and K+ issues, begins to increase osmotic pressure and cause fluids to move from peripheral tissues and interstitial fluid, this fluid in many food intolerants, has given them a bloated, Michelin man appearance, this oedema will begin to dissipate, once the recovery diet is adopted.

Some food intolerants don't retain fluid even before adopting the recovery programme, these people have often developed renal problems, and a slightly different approach has to be adopted with adrenal, liver, pancreas and kidney support, with the diet and herbs required to recover the situation, a qualified herbalist or naturapathic doctor should be consulted before this is approach undertaken.

The aforementioned problems cause only slight shifts in osmotic pressure, and intracellular extra cellular activity, these scenarios would not be recognised or evaluated as being a problem within the parameters of conventional medical tests, and therefore these shifts in pressure would never be considered as requiring treatment.

PLASMA CELLS AND IMMUNITY

Plasma cells are a vital link in immunity, if proteins are not being broken down to amino acids efficiently then the liver cannot assimilate or synthesise properly, plasma cells seek out malignant and foreign cells, and when encountered release enzymes which can destroy the offending cell.

If amino acids are in short supply, then the enzymes required for these processes to take place may not be produced efficiently, and consequently destruction of foreign cells is diminished.

Immunity is a very complex issue involving the following

• T lymphocytes

• B lymphocytes

• Memory T cells

• Cytotoxic T cells

• Helper T cells

• Memory B cells

• Plasma cells

• Antibody mediated immunity

• Acquired immunity

• Cell mediated immunity

So just to point out one deficiency in one cell type is a little presumptuous, but plasma cell activity appears to be one of the main problems encountered by food intolerants.
If these cells don't function properly it leaves us wide open to malignancy.

The whole immune system is suppressed in food intolerants, many of them easily catch colds and minor ailments and find them difficult to shrug off, again its due to the LIVER not having sufficient nutrients to assimilate and synthesise, to run these systems efficiently.

ACKNOWLEDGMENT

Dear John,

I would like to thank you for all your help regarding the flushes.

I would never have believed my liver could be so blocked, I've got rid of hundreds of stones and I've not finished yet, but I am well on the road to recovery and can eat a more varied diet.

I am getting more energy and beginning to enjoy life again. Thanks once again, I'll keep in touch.

Yours Faithfully

Roger Gilbert.

HERBAL TREATMENTS

HERBS USED TO RECOVER SYSTEMS?

The following herbs may be used to recover systems and alleviate symptoms, but these should not be self prescribed, it is better to see a qualified herbalist, or a naturopathic doctor, they will assess your health needs and prescribe accordingly, it is never as simple as just trying to recover one system, a holistic approach is required when herbs are used to treat a condition.

Liver herbs such as

● Barberry *berberis vulgaris*

● Fringe tree *chioanthus virginicus*

● Milk thistle *silibum marianum*

● Dandelion *taraxacum officionale* (not if aldosterone problems are present)

● Gentian *gentiana lutea*

Adrenal herbs such as:

● Liquorice *glycyrrhiza glabra*

● Borage *borago officianale*

● Sarsasparilla *smilax officianale*

Pancreatic herbs such as:

● Goats rue *galega officionale*

● Mountain grape *berberis aquifolium*

● Fringe tree *chioanthus virginicus*

Kidney herbs such as

● Stone root *collinsonia canadensis*

● Gravel root *eupatorium pupureum*

● Uva ursi *arctostaphylosa uva ursi*

● Hydrangea *hydrangea arborescens*

DARE I SAY IT...

If someone had said to me 30 years ago, I can give you a gallbladder and liver flush, to clean out your liver, or a kidney cleanse to clean out your kidneys, I would have said, absolute balderdash, you have to be operated on to remove gallstones or kidney stones.

I now know to my amazement and humility, that you can be very wrong in your perception of other methods of treatment.

Desperation, and the feeling of being driven into a dead end by the medical profession, where my illness was concerned, drove me; therefore I was forced into trying other methods and alternatives to alleviate my many symptoms.

This book and the treatments in it actually work, and have been arrived at after many highs and lows, and much experimenting and exasperation, after sometimes spending a wasted month or so, on some wild goose chase, whilst wading in the mire and mass of alternative treatments and concoctions.

It took sheer determination, and some of my friends say obsession, to see this intolerance phenomena to its final conclusion.

I have deliberated much before putting this chapter in my book, it's very easy to knock something, but I feel that many of the so-called alternatives are a little outlandish.

I have tried many other so-called alternative medicines and treatments, and found most of them to be ski/fi, some of these alternative medicine pundits arrive at the correct answer, and then proceed to go on into the realms of fantasy, and a complete obsession with outlandish beliefs, in some force field or some other irrational undertaking, this completely destroys their credibility in the eyes of many people, and therefore many of their very good treatments are enveloped, and lost, in the confusion and mire of the myriads of conflicting, misleading, and wrong information they feed to the general populous.

This is a dire shame, as many people could benefit from many of the so-called alternatives, and find relief from many minor illnesses, without resorting to medication, or even surgery.

Diet is the first and crucial factor in causing many minor ailments, and the medical profession would do well, to ask in the first instance, a patient with stomach problems or acid reflux, what do you eat? and give them in the first instance a healthy diet, instead of antacids or acid blockers, which in the long term only proceeds to compound the problem.

I could really get on my soap box about this subject, so I think I'd better leave it at that, before I get into deep water with the alternative community and others, whom I should thank, for they have helped a great deal in my recovery, after all that's where the gallbladder and liver flush, and the kidney flush came from.

So I apologise for any offence I may have caused to anyone in this chapter, but I felt that I had to voice my opinion, and at the end of the day, that is all it is, an opinion.

A LAST WORD

Mans profound intelligence often leads him to search for the complex when faced with a radical unsolvable problem, this on many occasions leads him astray, often the obvious is staring you in the face, but mankind inevitably takes numerous paths in his conquest for the actual, subsequently when an actual and truth is found it usually turns out to be very simple, and often the unexpected. And after you have arrived at a conclusion you then look back and say, how did it take this long to arrive at what now seems to be the obvious.

The saying "hindsight is the easiest thing in the world" springs to mind.

When the aspects of diet are related to the many illnesses and afflictions that are covered in this book, you can only arrive at one conclusion and make this radical statement. "A free unrestricted flow of bile enzymes and hormones from the liver and pancreas down through the entire common bile duct is, essential for the correct breakdown, absorption and interaction of vitamins minerals and nutrients required to sustain a healthy body".

So I say to those in the medical profession that the way wheat in particular, and sugar and dairy products to a lesser degree are processed is, a/or the causal factor of damage to the digestive tract and related organs in many people, and that there is not necessarily a measurable definable datum point to define a disease or condition.

So the only way to diagnose this condition is to study the life history of a person, and assess whether there is a possibility they could have become intolerant to wheat and dairy products, or as I've said many times before in this book processed and fortified wheat products, and pasteurised dairy products.

This condition I now know can have many symptoms, and these symptoms can vary from mild indigestion, to the many symptoms described in chapter 2.

It can be a very illusive condition to diagnose, and obviously a doctor just has not got the time in his busy day, and a ten-minute consultation, to properly assess the symptoms and diagnose this condition.

At the moment the medical profession use the antibody and flattened villi (small protrusion elements that line the intestine) test to define wheat intolerance, or to be more precise gluten intolerance, but patently this does not diagnose those of us who are intolerant to wheat and do not have these measurable scenarios, and therefore have no measurable definable datum point, and are thus left in medical no mans land, with little help, and are often made to feel like hypochondriacs, or a nuisance to the medical profession, and often put in the irritable bowel, I.B.S, or the M.E pigeonhole.

Over indulgence in these products over many years, patently culminates in the degradation of the digestive tract and related organs in those of us who are susceptible, but I now know there is a way back.

There is a very strong possibility that the majority of people with prolonged year on year stomach problems, have gained food intolerance, but only as a consequence of having a clogged liver and possibly gallstones, and will find relief from their symptoms and a new lease of life, if the measures detailed in this book are adopted.

Many inefficiencies, conditions and illnesses within the digestive tract are reversible if the measures in this book are adopted, without redress to medication.

I am now totally convinced that highly processed concentrated foods are the culprit, especially wheat protein (gluten), sugar and dairy products, if ingested in large quantities over a lengthy period of time.

Finally I hope this book has been of benefit to you and enabled you to discover a renewed enthusiasm and vigour for life, which may have been eluding you for many years, I thank you for purchasing this book, good luck and good health.

P.S

When you have fully recovered and regained your life, it would be very much appreciated if you would shout about this recovery programme from the rooftops.

If you come across anyone with the symptoms listed in this book, tell them about your experiences and help them in turn to regain their lives.

You are the best ambassador I have, and together we can help a significant proportion of the population to relieve themselves of this common affliction, and help to empty the doctors surgeries of people with lifelong stomach and bowel problems, throughout the world.

The common sense of one generation was always the new discovery to new generations.

He who gathers diligently, shall reap the rewards of his patience, for patience is a virtue, and virtuosity in itself breeds diligence, therefore he who gathers diligently.

Thank you

John Stephen Wrathall

NATURAPATHIC PRACTITIONERS

There are now many Naturopathic practitioners around Britain, and if you look on the internet you should be able to find one close to where you live.

They tend to have their specialities, dealing with treatments such as, homeopathy, acupuncture, diet, herbal, iridology, muscular skeletal, etc and use many different diagnostic techniques, to ascertain a diagnosis and treatment protocol.

● There are also practitioners in many other countries, the main overseas associations are listed below.

●The British Naturopathic Association, Somerset, England.

● Australian Naturopathic practitioners Association, Victoria, Australia.

● American Naturopathic medical Association, Pahrump Nevada, America.

● Canadian Association of Naturopathic Doctors, Toronto, Ontario, Canada,

For instance the local one I sometimes refer people to is,

Millennium Medicine Naturopathic Health
Room 3G
Garstang Business And Community Centre.
Garstang
Lancs
PR3 1EB
TEL 01995 605446

THANKS

I would like to thank the many people involved in the writing of this book, for their help and feedback, which enabled me to fully understand and arrive at the many conclusions regarding food intolerance; these include the following people or bodies.

Manchester University and the C.N.M, "College of naturopathic Medicine", for their extremely eye opening, in depth, informative, and interesting 4 yr course, on Naturapathic principles of Medicine, and other related studies.

- Janet Wrathall

- Richard Eccles.

- Linda Jackson

- Graham Bleasdale

- Andrew Singleton

- Bernard Cookson

- Robert Cornthwaite

- Patricia Colgan

- Mark Etherington

- John Billington

- Roger Gilbert

- Tyson printing, printing and binding of book.

- Dean Chillmaid @ Spacehopper Design, pagination and cover design.

Most of all thanks to my friends and acquaintances for putting up with me, through all the experiments and highs and lows, and the times I was not at available, due to university courses and other commitments.

John Stephen Wrathall, ND, Herb Dip.

INDEX

7

7 dehydrocholesterol, 180

A

a job interview or a stage appearance, 187

A, Bs, C, D, E, K, iron, zinc, selenium, folic acid, calcium, 204

aching gums, 87

Aching joints, 18

Aching muscles, 18

acid reflux, 20, 22, 25, 26, 38, 85, 88, 106, 116, 159, 260, 265, 268

acidic urine, 20

Acne, 18, 23, 25, 131, 173

adapted and evolved to eat, 96

ADH, 279, 280

Aesophogitis, 262, 265

aggressive and short fused, 93

albumins, 254, 277, 281

Alcohol is a toxin, 181

allergic, 52

allergy, 34, 52, 58

amino acid, 103, 129, 252, 256, 260, 274

Anaemia, 18, 22,39, 87, 131, 134, 203, 244, 262, 266, 268

anaemic, 140

anaphylactic shock, 52

angiotensinogen, 193, 254, 274, 275, 276, 277, 278, 279

antacids, 26, 106, 188, 202, 258, 268, 287

anti depressants, 202

antibiotics, 24, 26, 90, 162, 166, 269

antibody, 52, 91, 96, 108, 136, 151, 282, 288

anxiety,18, 87, 91, 131, 184, 185, 186, 188, 244, 261

Apple cider vinegar, 167, 169, 170, 172

Are we really that naïve, 216

arthritic, 18, 38, 132, 220

as a baby we are fed dairy products, 151

Aspartame, 70, 125

Athlete's foot, 18, 87, 92, 172

B

back in the same position, 96

Bacteria, 35, 37, 50, 72, 91, 97, 108, 129, 130, 148, 150, 157, 162, 165, 166, 167, 168, 170, 172, 180, 214, 263, 269

Bacteria can also invade the body, 172

barbecued foods, 180

Barley, 14, 42

beetroot, 15, 40, 48, 54, 60, 74, 77, 80, 92, 114, 218, 219, 222, 223, 226

Beetroot Cleanse, 80, 114, 218, 222, 223, 224

beriberi, 137, 134

binge drinking, 124, 180

bleeding gums, 87, 134

blind loop, 171

bloated, 18, 21, 25, 26, 28, 34, 35, 84, 85, 88, 89, 98, 107, 113, 129, 130, 131, 230, 258, 281

bloating, 11, 18, 22, 25, 26, 27, 36, 39, 72, 78, 86, 88, 89, 90, 91, 106, 131, 164, 229, 231, 234, 244, 261, 263, 265, 268

blood glucose levels, 126, 158, 159, 272, 273

blood sugar, 19, 38, 119, 125, 126, 127, 128, 132, 158, 159, 230, 272

blood tests and two biopsies, 38

brain, 88, 89, 185, 186, 187, 188, 189

Bran, 14, 15, 42, 49

Brandy, 70, 73

brothers or sisters, 27

Bruised feeling in stomach, 18

Bulgar, 14, 43

C

caffeine, 46, 76, 179

calcium, 36, 50, 103, 129, 138, 139, 140, 141, 144, 148, 149, 180, 218, 219, 221, 223, 277

candida, 20, 21, 35, 95, 100, 130, 133, 139, 150, 156, 162, 164, 169, 204, 207, 222, 231, 232, 244

Candida Albicans, 11, 48, 131, 139, 164, 222, 266

car fumes, 19, 180, 181, 183

catch 22 Scenario, 148, 204

celiac/celiac disease, 10,11, 19, 36, 38, 90, 96, 98, 101, 103, 108, 109, 110, 111, 112, 113, 118, 121, 131, 136, 137, 141, 142, 151, 168,

234, 244, 262, 263, 266, 269
chaff, 27, 39, 40, 80, 95, 120, 121, 122, 231, 232, 233, 234, 236, 237, 238, 239, 240, 241, 242, 244
change your mindset, 84
chlorine, 221
cholesterol, 100, 1,1, 103, 104, 115, 116, 120, 121, 123, 157, 180, 216, 235, 236, 237, 240, 242
Chorleywood process, 138
chronic fatigue, 20, 38, 100, 107, 137, 187, 196
cirrhosis of the liver, 180
cleaners, 180, 181
Coconut milk, 53, 54, 57, 71, 168, 170
coffee, 33, 70, 124, 179, 180, 181
coffee is an oxidiser, 70
Colofax, 202
Colon cancer, 131, 141
Colonitis, 109, 131, 245, 262, 266
constipation, 18, 21, 22, 23, 24, 51, 77, 85, 91, 92, 106, 107, 113, 116, 130, 150, 230, 256, 258, 259, 261, 263
Couscous, 14, 42
Cranberries, 15, 48, 72, 170
creatinine, 221
Crohn's disease, 22, 131, 141
Cystic fibrosis, 38

D
depression, 131, 185
dermatitis herpetiformis, 18, 38, 131
detergents, 19, 180, 183
detoxification and lymphatic system, 182
detoxify, 47, 55, 56, 70, 86, 92, 107, 112, 123, 124, 152, 169, 180, 181, 204, 222
Diabetes, 2, 11, 126, 127, 128, 131, 158, 159, 180, 272
diabetic, 2, 126, 127, 128, 158, 159, 228, 231, 238, 239, 272, 273
diagnose, 38, 91, 107, 109, 110, 112, 114, 150, 159, 191, 261, 288
Diarrhoea, 18, 22, 91, 169, 187, 188
digestive enzymes, 11, 15, 71, 72, 250
disturbed sleep, 20, 198, 265
diverticulitis, 22, 38 54, 55, 59, 109, 130, 132, 141, 234, 245, 262, 264, 266, 268

Drained of energy, 18, 21
dry patches of skin, 18, 21, 87, 93, 183
duodenum, 103, 105, 108, 112, 115, 116, 117, 118, 165, 189, 205, 237, 249, 250, 251, 252, 254, 256, 257, 259, 260
Durum, 14, 43, 142

E
elimination diet, 35, 36
emergency state, 22, 26, 47, 100, 107, 108, 110, 111, 112, 113, 118, 138, 164, 218, 263, 269, 272, 278
erection, 94
Escherichia coli, 172
Everything in moderation, 200
evolved or adapted, 214
evolved to eat, 86, 214
excessive sweating, 88
exhaustive tiredness, 189
extreme tiredness, 89

F
faecal test, 39, 270
fight or flight, 188
fingernails, 20, 21, 88, 93, 119, 230, 243
flour is bleached, 137
flush/flushed, 12, 42, 71, 72, 92, 95, 96, 106, 114, 118, 120, 121, 122, 124, 128, 167, 169, 178, 183, 197, 215, 219, 228, 229, 231, 232, 233, 234, 235, 236, 237, 238, 239, 240, 241, 242, 243, 244, 245, 246, 258, 262, 269, 273
folic acid, 76, 78, 79, 173, 204
fortified breads, 137
fried foods, 179, 180
fungal conditions, 174
fungal infections, 72, 88, 164, 172, 269
fungi that can affect your nails, 172
fungus, 171, 172

G
gallstones, 18, 19, 20, 26, 27, 39, 40, 47, 51, 72, 78, 79, 86, 92, 94, 108, 109, 111, 116, 117, 119, 120, 121, 124, 126, 127, 128, 132, 151, 169, 229, 230, 231, 232, 233, 234, 235, 236, 237, 238, 239, 240, 241, 242, 243, 244, 254, 259, 260, 287, 288
Garlic, 15, 48, 74, 51, 63, 65, 66, 67, 76, 77,

78, 79, 86, 167, 169, 170
Gin, 70, 73
Ginger, 14, 15, 43, 48, 71, 74, 55, 60
Give yourself some quality time, 199
glandular fever, 23
gliadin, 139, 142, 168
gluten, 10, 11, 14, 23, 25, 35, 36, 37, 38, 40, 42, 43, 46, 54, 56, 57, 58, 59, 62, 64, 65, 66, 67, 70, 76, 91, 96, 97, 98, 100, 109, 111, 113, 120, 121, 130, 136, 137, 138, 139, 141, 142, 143, 144, 151, 168, 218, 263, 288, 289
glycaemic index, 157
go on holiday abroad you feel better, 25
Gout, 88, 132, 141, 218, 220
gritty eyes, 86
Gums ache and bleed, 19
gut flora, 37, 77, 79, 94, 97, 100, 122, 126, 129, 130, 131, 150, 152, 157, 162, 164, 165, 166, 167, 168, 169, 170, 203, 263, 269

H
H.D.L, 100, 115, 127, 157 Haemorrhoids, 19, 261, 266
Headaches, 19, 85, 88, 92, 98, 132, 244, 264, 265
heart, 16, 48, 49, 101, 123, 200, 228, 278
Helicobacter pylori, 40, 76, 77, 90, 91, 107, 162, 205, 262, 266
herbal, 3, 53, 172, 202, 218, 219, 221, 222, 282, 286, 292
herbal cleanse, 40, 80, 114, 218, 219, 221, 222, 223, 224, 226
Herbal teas, 71
hospital, 10, 188, 243
household fridge, 215
hunter-gatherer, 213
hyperglycaemia, 126, 272
hyperglycaemic, 158
hypochondriacs, 288
Hypoglycaemia, 19, 22, 38, 88, 119, 26, 132, 230
hypoglycaemic, 128, 158, 272

I
I felt like a right plonker, 184
I have just described what is known as, 118
I.B.S, 10, 21, 22, 84, 91, 107, 110, 113, 118,

130, 132, 137, 186, 187, 244, 261, 262, 266, 269
if you fulfil the symptoms criteria, 12
ileum, 107104, 105, 134, 203, 249, 262, 269
Impotency, 19, 88, 94
impotent, 94
incompatible with our digestive tract, 216
indigestion, 20, 21, 116, 131, 258, 268, 288
insulin, 2, 99, 126, 127, 128, 158, 159, 272, 273
Intussusception, 243, 262, 266
iron, 18, 22, 37, 40, 78, 80, 107, 138, 140, 143, 145, 146, 149, 207, 208, 225, 271
Iron, 18, 22, 36, 39, 76, 77, 80, 103, 115, 130, 134, 137, 139, 140, 141, 144, 203, 204, 222, 262, 266, 268, 269, 279
islets of Langerhans, 127, 158, 272
It's absolutely crucial, essential, vital, and critical, 114
It's like an I.C.I chemicals plant, 122
Itchy rectum, 19, 85

J
jaundice, 119, 230
jejunum, 91, 103, 105, 109, 112, 140, 189, 202, 250

K
kidney, 16, 36, 37, 39, 40, 80, 87, 92, 100, 109, 110, 111, 112, 114, 118, 122, 123, 124, 129, 152, 167, 168, 169, 170, 180, 183, 188, 189, 217, 248, 262, 274, 286, 288
Kidney stones, 132, 149, 218, 219, 221, 222, 223, 225, 226, 287

L

L.D.L, 10, 115, 127, 157
Lactic acid, 50, 150, 168
lactobacillus, 150, 168
lactose, 37, 50, 76, 103, 129, 131, 148, 150, 152, 168, 263
late onset celiac disease, 111, 118, 234
leaky gut syndrome, 108, 110, 264
L-glutamine, 204
liver was clogged as a baby, 23
logical rational thought, 184
look at your own children, 27
look at your parents, 27
loose bowels, 18, 21, 22, 23, 24, 26, 36, 47, 70, 77, 85, 90, 92, 107, 108, 110, 111, 113, 117, 118, 130, 168, 187, 230, 237, 259, 261, 263, 265, 272
Lupus, 22
lymphatic system, 3, 108, 123, 172, 183, 229, 263

M

M.E, 10, 20, 21, 22, 100, 107, 114, 121, 137, 235, 277, 288
magnesium, 103, 141, 149, 218, 219, 221, 243, 244
man made oils, 180
Mango juice, 71
many intolerants are anaemic, 140
masked, 39, 86, 90, 288
masked by the bloating, 39
membranes, 115, 120
memory, 2, 91, 184, 187, 197, 245, 264, 282
Mentagrophytes, 172
milk thistle, 77, 124, 286
milled grain, 137
mind, 76, 91, 116, 120, 122, 179, 184, 185, 186, 187, 188, 189, 190, 197, 199, 288
molecular, 123, 144, 206, 209
more intolerant than their parents, 28
Myalgic encephalitis, 22, 38, 132, 262, 265, 266, 277
Mycobacterium vaginalis, 172

N

nervous situation, 187, 188
neurons, 68, 88, 189, 277
nicotinic acid, 137

O

oats will affect you, 138
Onions, 51, 55, 56, 60, 64, 65, 67, 76, 78, 79, 86, 167, 169, 170
Oregano, 66, 71, 77, 78, 169, 170
Osteoporosis, 132, 149
Our food is breaking down our digestive tract, 106
oxidants, 178, 179, 181, 182, 183

P

paint fumes, 180, 183
palpitations, 86, 93, 245, 264, 278
pancreas, 11, 38, 39, 70, 96, 99, 103, 105, 108, 114, 116, 122, 124, 125, 126, 127, 128, 130, 140, 158, 159, 166, 167, 180, 215, 236, 250, 251, 252, 254, 256, 259, 262, 268, 272, 273, 281, 288
pasteurising, 148
peristalsis, 94, 104, 107, 108, 110, 115, 116, 117, 118, 186, 202, 257, 259
pernicious anaemia, 134, 203, 262, 266, 268
PH, 105, 169, 172, 207, 252, 253, 254, 255, 256, 257, 259, 260, 261, 263, 264, 267, 270
phosphate, 218, 221, 224, 226
phosphorus, 138, 139
phytases, 139, 140
phytates, 139, 140
phytic acid, 14, 42, 96, 98, 138, 140, 141
Piles, 19, 87, 132, 261
potassium, 221, 276, 277, 279
Pre Menstrual tension, 132
pregnant, 127
preservatives, 28, 76, 125, 138, 181, 219
pro biotics, 14, 15, 44, 49, 50, 76, 77, 78, 150, 152, 168
Propionibacterium acnes, 177
Propolis, 77, 78, 167, 169, 170
Pseudamonas aeruginosa, 172
psychiatry, 190
pyramid, 206

R
refined sugar, 51, 96, 100, 121, 130, 148, 160, 171
rest is as important as exercise, 197
retention, 18, 85, 89, 91, 108, 111, 113, 131, 134, 229, 245
Rice milk, 53, 55, 58, 62, 72
Rickets, 133, 134, 137, 142
ridges on fingernails, 20
roseacea, 19, 23, 85
Russian roulette, 179
Rye, 14, 43

S
satisfied after eating, 189
scurvy, 134
selenium, 80, 204, 276
siblings, 27
Sinus problems, 132, 150
smoke, 19, 124, 179, 180, 182
smoking, 26, 179, 181
Smoking introduces lots of toxins, 181
sodium, 170, 221, 251, 252, 260, 276, 279
sore and dry throat, 92
sore throat, 20, 169
sourdough, 99, 139, 143
Soya, 14, 42, 45, 56, 70, 98, 138
spaced out, 20
Spelt, 14, 43, 143
spleen, 105, 124
sprays, 180, 181, 182
Staphylococcus aureus, 172
Stearic acid, 14, 45, 52, 76, 98, 205
stiff joints, 25, 95, 264
stomach, 3, 10, 14, 18, 20, 22, 23, 24, 27, 34, 35, 36, 40, 51, 68, 76, 77, 77, 78, 85, 88, 90, 92, 94, 102, 106, 107, 108, 115, 116, 117, 121, 123, 126, 134, 144, 162, 164, 179, 182, 186, 188, 192, 203, 205, 207, 229, 230, 233, 235, 238, 243, 244, 245, 249, 250, 256, 257, 258, 259, 261, 265, 287, 288, 290
Stomach ulcers, 101, 207
Stool colour, 73, 79, 94, 95
stop smoking, 26
Streptococcus pyogenes, 172
sugar, 2, 10, 11, 19, 23, 27, 28, 37, 38, 40, 46, 47, 50, 51, 54, 57, 61, 63, 68, 70, 76, 80, 96, 98, 99, 100, 103, 106, 109, 111, 113, 115, 119, 120, 121, 122, 123, 124, 125, 126, 127, 128, 129, 130, 132, 138, 148, 150, 151, 156, 157, 158, 159, 160, 165, 168, 171, 212, 218, 219, 230, 237, 260, 263, 272, 288
sulphate, 221, 243, 244
sweating, 20, 88, 217

T
take your pulse, 36
Tea is acidic, 70
thermostat, 192
thiamine, 36, 103, 134, 137, 189
thick toenails, 20, 88, 92, 164, 172
this is a revelation to them, 136
This overwhelms your ability to detoxify, 123
Thrush, 72, 132, 164, 168, 170, 207, 220, 222
thyroid, 22, 92, 96, 100, 112, 123, 129, 132, 141, 149, 169
Thyroid problems, 22, 100, 112, 132, 149
Tinea Pedis, 172, 260, 266
Tingling and numbness, 20
too much exercise, 196, 1971
toxic overload, 152, 182
toxins, 51, 71, 76, 86, 89, 92, 108, 112, 122, 124, 129, 143, 152, 167, 169, 178, 179, 180, 181, 182, 183, 185, 187, 204, 218, 222, 223, 224, 264
trigger intolerance, 12, 52
Triticale, 14, 44
Trychophyton, 172
Trychophyton Rubrum, 172

U
Ulcerative colitis, 22, 38, 101, 109, 132, 141, 234, 245, 262, 264, 266, 268
Ulcers, 40, 101, 108, 119, 132, 134, 162, 207, 230, 234, 245, 262, 264, 268
Unleavened bread, 143
urea, 221
Uric acid, 24, 218, 221, 224, 226
urinate, 92, 159
use this book as your bible of recovery, 12

V
V.L.D.L, 100, 115, 127
vast amounts of food to keep functioning,

113
vegetarian, 216
villi, 91, 96, 103, 108, 109, 110, 111, 118,
136, 141, 151, 252, 257, 260, 263, 288
vitamin B12, 203, 269
vitamin C, 98, 103, 134, 140, 167, 179, 202,
204
vitamin E, 14, 44, 76, 77, 78, 79, 140, 141,
202, 203, 204, 205, 239
Vodka, 70, 73

W
Warning 77, 91, 13, 162, 183, 225
water, 15, 18, 49, 57, 58, 60, 63, 65, 66, 72,
74, 89, 92, 103, 104, 111, 134, 142, 143, 170,
172, 217, 229, 223, 224, 225, 229, 238, 240,
242, 249, 251, 257, 259, 263, 276, 277, 287
weight will fall quite rapidly at first, 90
Whisky, 70, 73
without redress to medication, 106, 289

Y
yeast overgrowth, 16, 19, 20, 21, 23, 37, 38,
40, 46, 47, 48, 50, 51, 70, 71, 72, 76, 79, 80,
85, 86, 87, 87, 89, 92, 95, 100, 111, 119, 122,
126, 129, 131, 132, 148, 150, 152, 156, 162,
164, 165, 166, 167, 168, 169, 170, 171, 172,
204, 231, 232
yuppie flue, 10, 89

Z
zinc, 76, 78, 79, 86, 103, 204, 216, 270